Principles of
TOXICOLOGY

Karen E. Stine
Thomas M. Brown

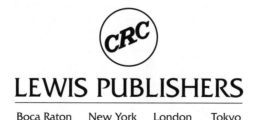

LEWIS PUBLISHERS

Boca Raton   New York   London   Tokyo

Contact Editor: Joel Stein
Project Editor: Albert W. Starkweather, Jr.
Marketing Manager: Greg Daurelle
Cover Designer: Denise Craig
PrePress: Kevin Luong
Manufacturing Assistant: Sheri Schwartz

Library of Congress Cataloging-in-Publication Data

Stine, Karen
    Principles of Toxicology / Karen Stine & Thomas M. Brown.
        p.   cm.
    Includes bibliographical references and index.
    ISBN 0-87371-684-1 (alk. paper)
    1. Toxicology I. Brown, Thomas M. (Thomas Miller)   II. Title.
RA1211.S75 1996
615.9—dc20   96-13905
                                                                                              CIP

© 1996 by CRC Press, Inc.
Lewis Publishers is an imprint of CRC Press.

No claim to original U.S. Government works
International Standard Book Number 0-87371-684-1
Library of Congress Card Number 96-13905
Printed in the United States of America   2 3 4 5 6 7 8 9 0
Printed on acid-free paper

DEDICATIONS

I would like to dedicate this to my husband, children, and parents in appreciation for all their support and encouragement.

K.E.S.

I wish to dedicate this effort to my many teachers, especially my parents, and the rest of my family.

T.M.B.

PREFACE

This book evolved from a course originally developed and taught at Clemson University beginning in the spring of 1987. In searching for a textbook to accompany this new principles of toxicology course, we discovered a need. Many of the available books were appropriate only as reference material for more advanced students; others were too narrowly focused one topic such as biochemical toxicology or ecological toxicology.

The purpose of this book is to serve as a comprehensive yet readable textbook for a first course in toxicology at the undergraduate or graduate level. We cover the broad and interdisciplinary field of toxicology through a "levels of organization" approach in presentation of this material. Initial chapters focus on molecular and cellular toxicology, the middle of the book stresses physiological toxicology, and the final chapters deal with environmental and ecological toxicology. Each chapter combines background material (to help students review and remember basic concepts) with new information in a manner which stresses principles and concepts. The book also contains extensive cross-referencing to unify the material.

We would like to thank all of our colleagues who contributed suggestions, comments, and their support to this project, as well as the editors and staff at CRC Press/Lewis Publishers who have helped make this book a reality.

THE AUTHORS

Karen E. Stine, Ph.D., is an Associate Professor and Director of the Toxicology Program in the Department of Biology/Toxicology at Ashland University in Ashland, OH.

Dr. Stine holds a B.S. in Physics and Biology from the College of William and Mary in Virginia, an M.S. in Environmental Science from the University of Virginia, and a Ph.D. in Toxicology from the University of North Carolina at Chapel Hill. She is a member of the Society of Toxicology, the Society of Environmental Toxicology and Chemistry, and the Council on Undergraduate Research.

At Clemson University, Dr. Stine codeveloped and cotaught a Principles of Toxicology course which was open to both undergraduate and graduate students. At Ashland University, she currently teaches an undergraduate Principles of Toxicology course, along with numerous other courses in the areas of toxicology and general biology. She has also authored or co-authored several research publications in the field of toxicology. Her research interests are in the area of mechanisms of toxicity, and currently focus on the role of stress proteins in cellular function and dysfunction.

Thomas Miller Brown, Ph.D. is Professor of Entomology at Clemson University where he teaches Toxicology of Insecticides, Principles of Toxicology, and Insect Biotechnology. He holds the B.S. from Adrian College and the Ph.D. from Michigan State University where he was introduced to the study of toxicology by Ronald E. Monroe and Anthony William Aldridge Brown. He is a member of the American Chemical Society, the International Society for the Study of Xenobiotics, and the Entomological Society of America. He has published on the biochemical toxicology of organophosphorus compounds and on the mechanisms of insecticide resistance in insects. He was Program Chairman of the ACS Special Conference "Molecular Genetics and Ecology of Pesticide Resistance". His current research on molecular genetics of resistance to insecticides includes formal research collaborations in Japan.

TABLE OF CONTENTS

1	MEASURING TOXICITY AND ASSESSING RISK

INTRODUCTION

Toxicology is the science of poisons, and has as its focus the study of the adverse effects of chemicals on living organisms. Although almost any substance in sufficient quantities (even water!) can be a poison, toxicology focuses primarily on substances which can cause these adverse effects when administered in relatively small quantities. Knowledge of the relative toxicity of substance is fundamental to all fields of toxicology, from development of a new drug, to the modeling of the effects of an environmental pollutant. This chapter describes approaches used by toxicologists to determine the toxicity of a substance. We consider principles of the dose vs. response relationship, methods used to evaluate toxicity in laboratory animals, and subsequent statistical analyses for quantitation of toxicity. We also discuss the use of toxicity data in assessing the risks of exposure to potentially hazardous substances.

TOXICITY TESTING METHODS

A wealth of information can be gathered from toxicity testing by carefully observing animals during and following exposure. These data may provide evidence for the mode of action of the substance and provide clues as to which physiological system, organs, and tissues could be affected.

Although specific protocols for toxicity testing have been developed by various regulatory agencies (such as FDA and EPA), they share many characteristics. Of course, in any study, the handling and treatment of animals must be the same for all animals in the study, whether they are in treated or control groups. Animals may be tagged for identification, using either simple numbered, metal *ear tags*, or more sophisticated devices such as electronic *transponding implants*. Animals must be housed in clean, comfortable conditions with access to adequate food and water. Typically, animals are housed in conventional, *box-type cages*, although in some cases specialized cages such as *metabolism cages* may be used. (These cages are equipped with a separator for collection and measurement of urine and feces, so that consumption of food and water can be measured more accurately.)

Daily or periodically, *weight* is typically determined, and animals are observed for *behavior* (comparing behavior of treated with control animals) and symptomology (such as tremors or convulsions, for example). During the exposure period, animals are monitored closely for symptoms of poisoning which might suggest the mechanism of poisoning of the substance. A slow onset of poisoning might suggest a *bioactivation* of the substance to a more toxic *metabolite*, or product, which accumulates as the parent substance is converted.

BIOACTIVATION
see also:
   Biotransformation   *Ch. 3, p. 21*

Following the exposure period, the animals are sacrificed and *necropsy* is performed. This is a procedure in which the treated and control animals are dissected and organs are weighed and examined for toxic effects in gross morphology and physiology. Sections of tissue samples may be sliced on a *microtome* and examined under the microscope for evidence of *histopathology* which is any abnormality in cell or tissue. Tissue samples may also be analyzed for the presence of biochemical indicators of pathology.

FACTORS TO BE CONSIDERED IN PLANNING TOXICITY TESTING

There are several questions which must be answered in determining the toxicity of a chemical substance. Among these are (1) through what physiological route does exposure occur (in other words, how does the substance get into the body), (2) how much of the substance is necessary to produce toxicity, and (3) over what period of time does exposure occur? Toxicity testing attempts to answer these questions and thus provide practical information about the risks involved in exposure to potentially toxic compounds.

Routes of Exposure

Various means of administration or *routes of exposure* are used in toxicity testing. *Oral toxicity* is of primary concern when considering a substance which might be ingested in food, such as the residue, or a pesticide or food additive, or taken orally as a drug. Dosing through the mouth is technically described as the *peroral* or *per os* (po) method. In some cases, the substance to be

ROUTES OF EXPOSURE
see also:
   Toxicokinetics   *Ch. 2, p. 11*

tested may be added directly to the animal's food or water. Alternatively, it may be dissolved in water, vegetable oil, or another *vehicle* (depending on the solubility of the test substance) and introduced directly into the esophagus or stomach through use of a curved needle-like tube (a process called *gavage*). Dermal administration may be considered for a substance which might be handled by workers, such as paints, inks, and dyes; or for cosmetics applied to the skin. The test substance is painted onto the skin, covered with a patch of gauze held with tape, and plastic is wrapped around the body to prevent ingestion of the substance. Finally, respiratory administration should be considered in testing industrial solvents or cosmetics applied in an aerosol spray.

Toxicity may also be assessed by direct injection of the substance, using a syringe and needle. *Intraperitoneal* (*ip*) injections are made into the body cavity; *intramuscular* (*im*) injections are placed into a large muscle of the hind leg; *subcutaneous* (*sc*) injections are placed just beneath the skin; *intravenous* (*iv*) injections are made directly into a large vein. Data derived from these injections are especially useful in the estimating doses for investigations of drugs which eventually may be injected by an analogous method in human patients.

Determining the Responses to Varying Doses of a Substance

Several terms are used to describe levels of exposure to toxicants. The terms dose and dosage have been used nearly interchangeably, although *dose* commonly refers to the amount of a chemical administered, and *dosage* refers to the amount of chemical administered per unit body weight of the recipient. Thus a dose of a drug might be expressed in milligrams while the dosage would be expressed as mg/kg body weight. In toxicity testing most chemical amounts are calculated and administered as dosages, which allows better standardization of the amount of chemical received, and allows a better basis for comparison of effects between individuals and species of widely varying body size. In respiratory exposures, exposure levels are usually measured by the concentration of the substance in the environment (in parts per million).

Quantitative toxicology involves challenging test animals with the substance to be evaluated which is applied in an ordered series of doses. The dose is controlled by the toxicologist; therefore, it is considered to be the *independent variable*. *Response* of the animals may be measured in many different ways, and is generally dependent on the dose applied (i.e., it is the *dependent variable*).

Responses can be scored and related to dose in order to determine the *dose vs. response relationship*. One response considered in toxicology is the death of the animal. This is scored as a *quantal value*, alive (no response: 0) or dead (response: 1), and recorded as *mortality*. A dose producing mortality is a *lethal dose* of the substance. In other experiments, the observed response may be a *continuous variable* which can be measured in each subject. Examples of continuous variables include consumption of oxygen, time to onset of convulsions, degree of inhibition of an enzyme, and loss of weight.

A basic principle of toxicology is that response varies proportionally to a geometric, not arithmetic, increase in dose. This means that to test a substance that produces responses in a small proportion of animals at 1 to 2 mg/kg, a geometric dosing range (1, 2, 4, 8, and 16 mg/kg) would be used rather than an arithmetic range (1, 2, 3, 4, and 5 mg/kg). Because of this, graphs relating dose and response are generally plotted with the response value on the y axis and the logarithm of the dose on the x axis.

Timing of Exposure

Often, the first of many considerations in toxicity testing is to assess the *acute toxicity* of the chemical. Acute toxicity is the toxicity which results from a single exposure to the substance. Typically, animals are dosed with a single dose and then observed for up to 14 days. One example of an acute toxicity test is the LD_{50}, which will be discussed later in this chapter. *Subacute toxicity testing* measures the response to substances which are delivered through repeated or continuous exposure over a period of time that generally does not exceed 14 days; *subchronic toxicity testing* involves repeated or continuous exposure over a period of 90 days. The final category of exposure is *chronic toxicity testing* which refers to repeated or continuous exposures which last for more than 90 days. To ensure sufficient challenge, animals are often exposed to the *maximum tolerated dose*, the greatest dose that neither kills nor causes incapacitating symptoms. While very high doses are used so that any chronic toxicity of the test compound will be observable, some experts consider that effects seen at large doses may be due to massive physical damage or *mitogenesis* (regeneration due to cell death), and thus may not accurately predict a substance's toxicity at lower doses.

THE LD_{50} EXPERIMENT

Testing

Traditionally, the *median lethal dose* has been used as a general measure of acute toxicity of any substance. This is the predicted dose at which one half of the individuals in a treated population would be killed. The median lethal dose is determined by exposing groups of uniform test animals to a geometric series of doses of the substance of interest under controlled environmental conditions. The abbreviation LD_{50}, for lethal dose 50, is often used for the median lethal dose. The standard laboratory animal used in this test is the white Norway rat, *Rattus norwegicus*.

The dose is expressed in *dosage units* of milligrams of active ingredient of the test substance administered per kilograms of body weight of the test organisms (mg/kg). The highest dose administered in a typical LD_{50} experiment is chosen so that 90% or more of the animals in the highest dose group will be killed. The choice of the highest dose can be estimated from previous results with chemically similar substances, or by a pilot, range-finding experiment in which a smaller number of animals are exposed to a wide range of dilutions. Then *serial dilutions* of that dose are used to produce a gradient of intermediate responses over four or five doses. Typically, at least 10 animals (ideally, 5 males and 5 females) are exposed at each of 6 doses plus there is a *negative control* group exposed only to the vehicle.

In LD_{50} determinations, the test substance is usually applied as *technical grade*, the practical grade as manufactured for sale and use (usually of approximately 95% purity). In some cases, an agency might require additional tests with the *analytical grade* (which is greater than 99% pure). If necessary, a sample can be tested by *gas chromatographic* or *high performance liquid chromatographic analysis* to verify the purity. A vehicle and route of administration must be chosen, based in part on the *physical properties* of the test substance including solubility in water, organic solvents, and corn oil; melting point, boiling point, and vapor pressure; and color and odor.

To perform the dosing, animals are chosen to be of similar weight, fasted overnight, numbered, and then assigned to treatment groups from a table of random numbers. Doses are applied beginning with the negative control, which is vehicle only, and then increasing doses of the test substance. (In this way, the same syringe can be used with no risk of contaminating a lower dose with the residue of a higher dose.) For each dose, a solution is prepared so that a small volume of vehicle, (e.g., 2.0 ml), will contain the intended dose when administered to the animal of average size. For example, if a dose of 10 mg/kg is intended, and the average rat weighs 200 g (0.2 kg), then the concentration of the test substance in oil solution should be 1.0 mg/ml. If the subject rat weighs 200 g, then 2.0 ml administered will result in the intended dose of 10 mg/kg. If the next rat weighs only 190 g, then the amount administered can be reduced to 1.9 ml to maintain the desired dose of 10 mg/kg.

Analysis

In any population, a very small proportion of individuals are very *susceptible* while another very small proportion of individuals are very *tolerant* to the same dose of the same poison. Some variability is actually *experimental error* due to such factors as the precision in administering the dose, environment of the animal, condition of the animal such as fasting, handling of the animal, etc. True heterogeneity is due to the *genetic variability* in physiological characteristics of the animals (although it is expected that inbred strains of rodents used in laboratory experiments would be much less heterogeneous in response than wild populations of the same species).

This variation in response is observed as the long "tails" of the dose vs. response histogram (Figure 1). If tolerances of individuals are *normally distributed* in the population of rats tested (as commonly assumed), then a *sigmoid curve* would describe the accumulated percentage mortality plotted vs. the logarithm of the dose (Figure 2). The increasing mortality observed at each higher dose is the

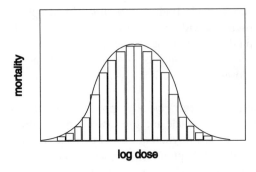

Figure 1
Histogram of normal distributed responses to a substance.

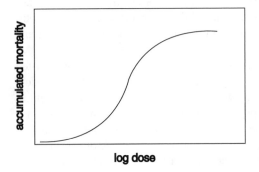

Figure 2
Accumulated responses (sigmoid curve).

result of accumulating responses of lesser tolerant to more tolerant individuals in each group.

The median lethal dose is often calculated by transforming the accumulated percentage mortality at each dose to a *probit mortality score*. This is a type of probability transformation in which one *probit unit* is defined as being equal in magnitude to one standard deviation unit of the response. Probit mortality scores plotted vs. the logarithm of the dose will produce a straight line from which the median lethal dose can be predicted (Figures 3 and 4). The *slope* of the probit plot line is related to the uniformity of response within the animal population. If the slope of the response were 2.0, a rather typical value, then approximately 68% of the population would be expected to respond to a ten-fold range in doses centered at the median lethal dose. On the other hand, if the slope of the response were 6.0, then more than 99.6% of the population would be expected to respond to a ten-fold increase in dose centered at the median lethal dose. An extremely homogeneous response was observed in CF1 mice exposed to an organophosphorus agent; there was a change of 18.8 probit units of response per 1.0 $\log_{10}$ increase in dose (Figure 4).

Alternative Tests

Although the median lethal dose is traditionally a very important value for toxicologists to use when considering the toxicity of a substance, this experiment has been criticized increasingly because of the large number of animals needed to

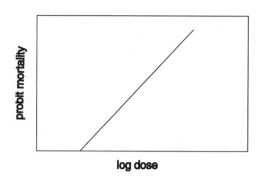

Figure 3
Log dose vs. probit transformed
responses.

gain a rigorous estimate. If a less precise estimate of the median lethal dose is acceptable, then a substitute called the *up-and-down method* which requires fewer animals can be used. This method was developed to find optimum mixtures of explosive materials with fewer trials and less waste and hazard. In the method, one animal is exposed to one dose of the substance. If it survives, then a second animal is exposed to a higher dose. If the second animal survives, another higher dose is administered until mortality is observed. Following mortality, the next animal is exposed to a lower dose and following survival, the next animal is given a higher dose, until an "equilibrium" is observed.

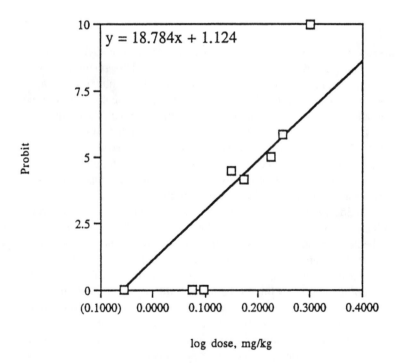

Figure 4 Mortality of CF1 mice exposed to 4-nitrophenyl methyl(phenyl)phosphinate.

From less than ten animals, the population median lethal dose can be estimated by the up-and-down method with similar accuracy to the full scale experiment exposing more than 60 animals. One deficiency of this test is that the variability of response cannot be estimated. Another disadvantage is the extra time required in waiting to score one animal before determining the dose for the next animal; however, this problem can be partially solved by reducing the observation period. Despite these problems, for most routine purposes of comparing the toxicity of poisons, the up-and-down method will provide sufficient information while sacrificing far fewer animals.

Categories of Toxicity

A somewhat arbitrary system of toxicity ranking has evolved based on the median lethal dose of a substance. A substance with a median lethal dose less than 1 mg/kg is considered to be "extremely toxic," while various definitions of "highly toxic," "moderately toxic," and "slightly toxic" have been proposed. Generally, "highly toxic" substances have a median lethal dose of less than 50 mg/kg, "moderately toxic" have a median lethal dose of less than 500 mg/kg, and "slightly toxic" have a median lethal dose of greater than 500 mg/kg and up to approximately 5 g/kg which approaches the practical limit of most dosing techniques.

MIXTURES

Mixtures of poisons can be more toxic or less toxic than predicted from the toxicity of the individual components of the mixture. This phenomenon of increased toxicity of a mixture is known as *synergism* and it results from an interaction of one component with the pharmacokinetics or pharmacodynamics of the second component; e.g., the first component might interfere with the elimination of the second component so that a given exposure of the second component produces higher concentrations in the body when applied in the mixture. *Antagonism* is the observation of less than predicted toxicity from a mixture; e.g., when one component induces a higher rate of inactivation of the second component resulting in a higher concentration of a less toxic metabolite.

Drugs, pesticides, industrial chemicals, etc. when used in mixtures, or when giving simultaneous exposure, should be evaluated empirically for interactions to determine whether there is synergism or antagonism. When one component is nontoxic, this test is relatively simple; the nontoxic component can be administered at a high concentration with the complete range of doses of the toxic component. If the dosage–mortality line of the mixture differs significantly from the dosage–mortality line of the toxic component alone, then an interaction is indicated. If both components are toxic, then the test for an interaction is more complex. One approach is to prepare a mixture containing each component at its median lethal dose. Dilutions are made and administered; then the observed dosage–mortality line is compared to a line predicted by adding the expected mortalities for the individual components at each dilution.

TOXICITY, HAZARD, AND RISK

Toxicity and Hazard

Keep in mind that an estimate of toxicity is not a direct estimate of hazard. For any substance, the term *hazard* can be used to describe the actual risk of poisoning. Toxicity is only one variable to be considered in predicting how hazardous a substance will be during practical use. Another significant variable which must be considered is potential level of human exposure to the substance. This must be predicted based on factors such as the concentration and circumstances of use of the substance. While the intrinsic toxicity of a substance cannot be altered because it is a basic property of that substance, it is possible to reduce hazard of a toxic substance by reducing the practical risk of exposure. A simple example is the invention of *childproof packaging* of nonprescription drugs which reduces the hazard associated with some drugs by making access to the drug more difficult. In another example, hazards posed by pesticides to the pesticide applicator have been reduced by preparing the pesticide in *dissolvable polymer bags* containing premeasured quantities designed to be dropped into the sprayer tank without opening. This innovation greatly reduced the risk of exposure to formulated pesticide concentrates by eliminating measuring and mixing by the applicator.

The Role of Testing in Estimation of Hazard

Toxicological data from laboratory studies such as those described here are often used by regulatory agencies in the attempt to estimate the hazard to human health posed by a particular toxicant. Along with laboratory data, data from *epidemiological* studies are also used in risk estimation. These studies examine the relationships between exposure to a toxicant (usually accidental or voluntary exposure) and either disease *incidence* (the rate at which new cases of the disease appear in a human population) or disease *prevalence* (the number of existing cases of the disease at a particular point in time).

It can be quite difficult to extrapolate from laboratory and epidemiological studies to real world situations, which is why the processes of risk assessment and management are often fraught with controversy. Although laboratory animals can serve as models for humans in toxicological testing, species differences do exist. Also, many scientists have criticized the practice of using very high doses of toxicants during laboratory testing and then attempting to apply the results to a situation where human exposure levels are actually very low.

Epidemiological studies have some drawbacks, however. Because of variability in genetic and environmental factors between individual humans, it can be extremely difficult to be sure that differences in disease incidence or prevalence between exposed and control groups are really due to the factor being tested and not to some other *confounding factor*. Also, exposure levels may be difficult to estimate (particularly if exposure to the toxicant occurred some time in the past). To maximize reliability of results, exposed and control groups are often matched as closely as possible for potential confounding factors such as age, sex, lifestyle factors, working conditions, or living conditions. Also, the larger the number of individuals participating in the study, the easier it is to detect small differences between the exposed and control groups.

Risk Assessment and Risk Management

In the process of *risk assessment*, hazard is weighed against benefit as regulatory decisions are made concerning potentially toxic substances. The National Academy of Sciences/National Research Council published a report in 1983 outlining the steps involved in risk assessment and risk management. They identify four main components of the process of risk assessment: (1) *hazard identification*, where it is determined whether or not a substance is a potential health hazard; (2) *dose–response evaluation*, where the dose–response relationship is quantified; (3) *exposure assessment*, where potential exposure levels are estimated; and (4) finally, this information is merged in the process of *risk characterization*, where effects on the exposed population are estimated. Descriptions of risk are often phrased in terms of the chances of contracting a particular disease during a lifetime of exposure to a particular toxicant at a given level of exposure.

Risk assessment is then followed by *risk management*, which is the process by which regulatory decisions are made concerning health risks. Risk management takes not only risk assessment results, but also other political, social, and economic factors into account when making decisions about regulating potential toxicants. Government agencies involved in risk management include the Occupational Safety and Health Administration (OSHA), the Food and Drug Administration (FDA), and the Environmental Protection Agency (EPA).

REFERENCES

Beck, B. D., Calabrese, E. J., and Anderson, P. D., The use of toxicology in the regulatory process, in *Principles and Methods of Toxicology*, Hayes, A. W., Ed., Raven Press, New York, 1989, chap. 1.

Bruce, R. D., An up-and-down procedure for acute toxicity testing, *Fund. Appl. Toxicol.*, 5, 151, 1985.

Joly, J. M. and Brown, T. M., Metabolism of aspirin and procaine in mice pretreated with *O*-4-nitrophenyl methyl(phenyl)phosphinate or *O*-4-nitrophenyl diphenylphosphinate, *Toxicol. Appl. Pharmacol.*, 84, 523, 1986.

Morton, M. G., Risk analysis and management, *Sci. Am.*, July 1993, 32.

Scala, R. A., Risk assessment, in *Casarett and Doull's Toxicology*, Amdur, M. O., Doull, J., and Klaassen C. D., Eds., Pergamon Press, New York, 1991, chap. 31.

2 TOXICOKINETICS

INTRODUCTION

Interactions of a poison with an organism can be considered in three phases: *exposure*, *toxicokinetics*, and *toxicodynamics*. During the *exposure phase*, contact is established between the poison and the body via one or more routes, e.g., a volatile air pollutant inhaled into the body. Then, during the *toxicokinetic phase*, the poison undergoes movement (Greek: *kinesis*) through the body. This movement includes absorption into the circulatory system, distribution among tissues (including those which will serve as sites of action), and then elimination from the body. The *toxicodynamic phase* is the exertion of power (Greek: *dynamos*) of the poison through its actions on affected target molecules and tissues. These phases can be overlapping so that once exposure occurs, all phases of action can be in effect simultaneously in the body.

The principles of toxicokinetics, like most principles of toxicology, are derived from the science of *pharmacology*, which is the study of the action of drugs. Toxicology and pharmacology are naturally related because while most drugs are *therapeutic* (medicinally effective) over a narrow range of doses, they are also *toxic* at higher doses. In fact, many clinically important drugs are moderately toxic; therefore, they must be administered very carefully to avoid reaching toxic concentrations in the body.

A very practical problem in pharmacology is encountered in determining how to administer repeated doses of a drug in order to maintain the proper therapeutic concentration in the bloodstream. To avoid toxicity, the physician must understand how the concentration changes to predict the amount of the dose and the interval between doses. This problem and other related problems are the subject of *pharmacokinetics*.

The principles of pharmacokinetics apply to toxic substances as well as to drugs. In *toxicokinetics* one might want to estimate how concentrations of a toxicant may change over time. For example, one might want to see whether a toxicant is quickly excreted or whether repeated exposures will lead to accumulation in the body. There are, however, often differences in chemical properties between drugs and other types of toxicants which can produce differences in toxicokinetics. There are several environmentally important toxic substances (such as some pesticides, for example) which have high levels of *lipophilicity* (solubility in lipid) and high levels of *persistence* (due to slow degradation rates). These properties result in very slow toxicokinetics when compared to most pharmaceuticals. Many common drugs may be absorbed, exert an effect, and be eliminated in hours or even minutes. By contrast, some lipophilic substances found in the environment may be very slowly *accumulated*, and once exposure is terminated, they may be very slowly eliminated over days or months.

This chapter examines principles of absorption, distribution, and excretion of toxicants and looks at some simple mathematical models used to study the way toxicants enter, move through, and exit the body.

ABSORPTION

There are several possible routes of absorption for toxicants. What all routes have in common is that they present a cellular barrier which toxicants must cross to enter into the bloodstream. Thus, toxicants which can easily cross cell membranes (through simple diffusion or other transport processes) can be more easily absorbed than toxicants which cannot. The primary chemical property that enhances the ability of a toxicant to diffuse across biological membranes is *lipophilicity* (the ability to dissolve in lipids such as the phospholipids which make up the bulk of the membrane). Other properties that aid in diffusion include *small size* (which allows the toxicant to fit more easily between membrane molecules) and *neutral charge* (which allows the toxicant to avoid interactions with charged groups on membrane molecules).

The three major routes of absorption for toxicants are oral, respiratory, and dermal. Other routes include various sites for injection such as *intramuscular*, *intraperitoneal* (into the peritoneal cavity), *intravenous*, or *subcutaneous*.

The Oral Route of Absorption

One common route of absorption for toxicants is the *oral* route. Absorption can occur all along the gastrointestinal tract from the mouth to the large intestine. One factor which influences the site of absorption is the time a toxicant spends in that region. Thus, little absorption usually occurs in the mouth because of the limited time a toxicant spends there, while the much longer time it takes a toxicant to move through the small intestine gives plenty of opportunity for absorption. Also, surface area of the region is a factor, as is pH. Some toxicants tend to *ionize*, which is to gain or lose electrons and thus become negatively or positively charged ions. *Weak bases* ionize in low pH environments, while *weak acids* ionize in high pH environments. Because ionization decreases likelihood of absorption, weak bases are more likely to be absorbed in the higher pH found in the small intestine, while weak acids are more likely to be absorbed in the lower pH found in the stomach. When all factors are considered, as is the case with absorption of nutrients from food, most absorption of toxicants occurs in the small intestine.

The small intestine has a high surface area, a neutral pH of approximately 6, and is highly vascularized (contains many blood vessels). Most toxicants cross the epithelial cells lining the small intestine and enter the bloodstream by diffusion, although some enter through specific transport mechanisms such as *active transport* or *facilitated diffusion*. Active transport and facilitated diffusion both require the participation of protein carriers within the membrane and are generally quite limited in the molecules which they can carry. Thus, toxicants which can enter through these mechanisms are generally those which are structurally quite similar to the molecule normally moved by the carrier. For example, heavy metals such as lead may enter through the transporter which normally carries calcium.

Typically, a portion of an orally administered drug or toxicant will be unavailable for absorption into the general circulation. Some of the substance will simply continue through the alimentary tract. Factors which can influence absorption include presence or absence of other material in the gastrointestinal tract, the presence or absence of disease, and age of the individual. Also, since blood from the lower gastrointestinal tract travels through the *portal vein* to the liver prior to traveling to the rest of the body, a portion of the substance may be metabolized and deactivated in the liver prior to reaching other tissues. This phenomenon is known as the *first-pass effect*, which means that some drugs or toxicants may have less of an effect when administered orally than when administered through another route.

Respiratory Route of Absorption

Another important route of absorption is through the respiratory system. Inhaled gases pass through the nose, pharynx, larynx, trachea, and bronchi prior to entering the lungs. Water-soluble *gases* tend to be absorbed in the watery mucus which lines the upper part of the respiratory tract, while less water-soluble gases continue into the lungs. With *particles*, size is the determining factor. Large particles are screened out by cilia and mucus in the upper part of the tract, while smaller particles

ABSORPTION OF GASES AND PARTICLES
see also:
Respiratory toxicology   *Ch. 7, p. 95*

continue into the lungs for absorption. In the lungs, barriers to diffusion are few, because the cells which line the lungs are thin and located in very close proximity to blood vessels.

Dermal Route of Absorption

Of the three major routes, the dermal route of absorption provides the greatest cellular barrier. The skin consists of an epidermal layer made up of many layers of epithelial cells, and a dermal layer made of connective tissues. Because blood vessels are located in the dermal layer, a toxicant must pass through the epidermis first. The top layer of epidermal cells provides the greatest barrier to diffusion, because these cells not only have thickened cell membranes but are also filled with a protein called *keratin*. These modifications effectively block all but the most lipid-soluble substances from penetrating farther into the epidermis or dermis. Factors which influence dermal absorption include differences in thickness and degree of keratinization between skin in different body regions, and the condition of the skin. Injuries (e.g., scrapes, burns, cuts) which remove the keratinized layer of epithelial cells can increase significantly the potential for dermal absorption.

DISTRIBUTION

When a drug is administered intravenously at a known dose, it is assumed to be instantaneously dissolved in the blood or plasma. Plasma can then be sampled immediately upon administering the dose and at intervals after dosing. The concentrations of the toxicant in the plasma are measured and the concentration at time zero can be found by extrapolation. The *volume of distribution* of the toxicant is found by dividing the amount of drug in the body (the total amount of drug administered, in milligrams), by the concentration in plasma at time zero. If all the drug remained in the plasma, this volume of distribution would be equal to the volume of plasma (which for a 70-kg human is approximately 3.0 L). For example, if 3 mg were administered to a 70-kg human, and the concentration at time zero were 1.0μg/mL, then the volume of distribution would be 3.0 L (or 0.043 mL/kg).

Frequently, however, the value for volume of distribution of a drug or toxicant exceeds the volume of plasma in the body. This indicates that some of the drug or toxicant has left the plasma and has entered the fluid between and within the cells. Thus volume of distribution gives an indication of the ability of a drug or toxicant to leave the bloodstream and distribute into the tissues.

The rate at which a drug or toxicant is distributed to the various tissues of the body depends on several factors. Chief among these is the rate at which blood is supplied to the tissue. Tissues with a high *rate of perfusion* (rate of blood flow) such as the heart, liver, and kidney will thus also have a high rate of delivery of toxicants.

BLOOD-BRAIN BARRIER
see also:
   Neurotoxicology   *Ch. 9, p. 119*

There are some tissues, however, which have anatomical and physiological modifications that act to limit the delivery of toxicants. The tissues of the central nervous system, for example, are protected by a system known as the *blood-brain barrier*. This "barrier" is a result of tighter junctions between cells that make up the capillaries in the central nervous system, as well as the wrapping of capillaries in a cellular "blanket" that increases the width of the cellular barrier to diffusion that toxicants must cross. As a result, only highly lipid-soluble toxicants have easy access to the central nervous system.

There are some tissues with high affinity for certain toxicants, so that toxicants may accumulate there to high levels. Some toxicants bind to plasma proteins such as *albumins*. This tends to hold the toxicant in the bloodstream and delay release to other tissues. Liver and kidney contain proteins called *metallothioneins* which bind and hold heavy metals such as cadmium and zinc. Heavy metals may also accumulate in bone, and highly lipid soluble compounds (such as DDT) can accumulate in fat tissues. The tissues where toxicants accumulate are sometimes referred to as *storage depots*.

ELIMINATION

Elimination is the loss of the parent drug or toxicant from the body due to *biotransformation* of the parent drug, **A**, to *metabolites*, **B** or **C**, and also from *excretion* of the parent drug in urine or feces.

BIOTRANSFORMATION
see also:
Biotransformation *Ch. 3, p. 21*

Metabolites are products of chemical changes in the drug which are catalyzed by various enzymes in the body. These products may vary in toxicity and therapeutic effect from the parent drug. When biotransformation results in a less toxic product, the process is *detoxication*; however, some reactions form more toxic products from the parent and are known as intoxication or *bioactivation* reactions.

The major route of excretion of most drugs and toxicants is through the kidneys. Drugs or toxicants and/or their metabolites are filtered from the blood and excreted in the urine. Other drugs and toxicants and/or their metabolites may be removed from the blood by the liver, excreted into the bile, and eliminated through the gastrointestinal tract. Other routes of elimination include through the respiratory system, or through secretions such as saliva, sweat, or milk.

TOXICOKINETIC MODELS

Mathematical Models of Elimination

Many common drugs and toxicants are water soluble and they are carried through the body in the blood. The blood-borne concentration can be measured by chromatographic analysis of a small sample of blood. Administration of a drug or toxicant is followed by very rapid absorption into the blood (which results in increasing concentration), and the slower elimination of drug from the body (which causes the concentration in the blood to decline). These processes can be mathematically modeled, and the elimination rate can be used to predict drug or toxicant concentrations.

Absorption and elimination are opposite processes, and as such, they cannot be estimated when both are in operation. To measure elimination from the blood without needing to take into account adsorption, a drug or toxicant can be injected intravenously. In a typical experiment the drug or toxicant is introduced into a large vein of a rat by injection in a small volume of carrier. Assuming that the drug or toxicant has a high solubility in water, it will dissolve throughout the blood almost instantaneously and thereafter will decline in concentration. Repeated sampling of blood and measurement of the declining concentrations with time will then allow the elimination kinetics to be determined.

The rate of elimination of a drug, where $[A^b]$ is the concentration of the drug, **A**, in the body, can be described mathematically as:

$$\Delta[A^b_t]/\Delta t$$

The rate of elimination bears units such as: $mg*kg^{-1}*min^{-1}$, or $mg*kg^{-1}*hr^{-1}$.

For some drugs or toxicants the rate of loss from the body is constant over time, independent of the concentration of the drug in the body. In this case the elimination is described as a *zero-order* kinetic process (Figure 1). In practice, few drugs are eliminated in a zero-order process. One that is, however, is ethanol. Although unusual, ethanol pharmacokinetics are very important due to the common problem of excess alcohol drinking. Unfortunately, a high dose of ethanol will not be eliminated at a higher rate than a normal dose because the elimination rate is independent of the concentration in the body. For the *zero-order* process, since **A** will be eliminated at the same rate continuously, even as the concentration declines, the equation becomes:

$$\Delta[A^b_t]/\Delta t = -K_0$$

where K_0 is called the *zero-order elimination rate constant*. Knowing the concentration of the drug in the body at any given time, $[A^b_t]$, and the rate of elimination (in the case of zero-order kinetics, $-K_0*\Delta t$), the concentration at a later time, t+x, can be predicted by the equation:

$$[A^b_{t+x}] = -(K_0 * \Delta t) + [A^b_t]$$

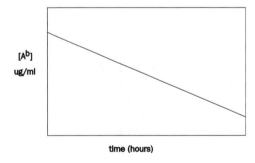

[A^b]
ug/ml

time (hours)

Figure 1
Zero-order process of elimination

The time required to eliminate a given portion of the drug via a zero-order process will vary and will lengthen as the initial concentration is increased.

If the rate of elimination of a drug or toxicant is first very rapid, and then becomes less rapid with subsequent sampling, it might follow a *first-order* process of elimination. The first-order process is observed as a logarithmic decay in the concentration of drug in the body in which the rate of loss is dependent on the concentration of the drug in the body, $[A^b_t]$ (Figure 2). The mathematical relationship describing first-order elimination kinetics is:

$$\Delta[A^b_t]/\Delta t = -K[A^b_t]$$

in this case, the *proportion* (not the amount) of the drug lost per unit time is constant. The exponential change in the concentration in the body is a constant value, the *first-order elimination rate constant*, **K**. Units of **K** are per time, such as min^{-1}, or hr^{-1}.

To predict the concentration of the drug after a period of time, you can use the equation:

$$\ln[A^b_t] = -K * t + \ln[A^b_0]$$

where $[A^b_0]$ is the initial concentration of **A** in the plasma. This equation may be more useful in the following form, in which the natural log (ln) has been converted to the base 10 log (log):

$$\log[A^b_t] = (-K * t)/2.303 + \log[A^b_0]$$

This equation takes the form of a straight line if you plot the log $[A^b_t]$ vs. time (Figure 3). (An easy way to do this is to use semilogarithmic paper which makes the logarithmic conversion for you automatically.) The slope of this line is $-K/2.303$.

Most drugs are eliminated in a process that resembles first-order pharmacokinetics; however, in practice, the process is usually more complicated. Rather than behaving as if the body were only one single *compartment*, most drugs and

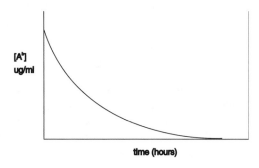

Figure 2
First-order process of elimination,
arithmetic plot.

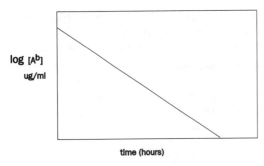

Figure 3
First-order process of elimination, logarithmic plot.

toxicants actually move between multiple body compartments. Typical experimental results suggest that there may be two, three, or even more first-order processes by which the drug is eliminated. This would correspond to a body containing several compartments, each eliminating the drug by a slower first-order process. As described above, the first-order elimination constant from a single compartment can be determined simply from the log concentration vs. time plot of the observed data. When a multicompartment model is necessary, then only the final rate constant, representing loss from the slowest compartment, can be determined directly from a plot. Prior to final elimination, the observed data represent simultaneous loss from multiple departments and faster processes must be estimated by working back from the final compartment by a more complex mathematical modeling process.

Clinical administration of drugs in a multiple-dose regimen requires the estimation of drug *clearance* which is the volume of blood or plasma which would be cleared (purged) of the drug per unit time to account for the elimination of the drug. Total systemic clearance is simply the *dose* (e.g., in mg*kg^{-1}) divided by the *area under the plasma-concentration-vs.-time elimination curve* (*AUC*) for that dose (generally expressed as mg*ml^{-1}*min).

$$\text{clearance} = \text{dose} / \text{AUC}$$

Thus, the typical value for clearance is given in units of ml*min^{-1}*kg^{-1}. Considering that AUC is inversely related to clearance, we see that for two drugs administered at identical doses, the one with the smaller AUC will have a larger value for clearance.

Absorption and Bioavailability

However, not all drugs or toxicants are administered intravenously, and methods do exist to quantify rates of absorption. For typical drugs or toxicants, absorption from the gut is a faster process than elimination. Thus, the concentration of the drug in the blood will initially depend on both the absorption and elimination rates and will rise rapidly to some peak concentration at which rate of absorption is equal to rate of elimination. Concentrations will then fall again, as elimination becomes the dominating process (Figure 4). Because absorption and elimination are simultaneous processes from an oral dose, it is more accurate and far simpler to estimate an elimination rate from the i.v. experiment described above rather than attempting to derive it from an oral dose experiment. From the elimination rate, and the data obtained in the oral dose experiment, the absorption rate can be determined also.

The AUC when the blood concentration of a drug or toxicant is plotted vs. time can also be used to estimate drug *bioavailability*. Bioavailability describes the extent to which a drug or toxicant is absorbed orally as compared to intravenous administration and is defined as:

$$(AUC_{oral} / dose_{oral}) / (AUC_{i.v.} / dose_{i.v.})$$

The closer this number is to 1, the better the absorption of the compound through the oral route.

CONTRASTING KINETICS OF LIPOPHILIC SUBSTANCES

Many xenobiotics are of interest to toxicologists because they are slowly eliminated and accumulate in the body. Such compounds, when administered in the experiments typical of pharmacokinetics as described above, sometimes have very large volumes of distribution and very low clearance values. A recent example is the new anthelmintic veterinary drug, *ivermectin*, which is given prophylactically for dog heartworm. This drug is eliminated very slowly and can be measured in the plasma after many days. These slow pharmacokinetics are very beneficial in that the drug is efficacious with administration only once per month, while older alternatives must be administered daily which is very inconvenient.

With some very lipophilic xenobiotics, the simple one-compartment model is not realistic because there is poor solubility in plasma and high solubility in body lipids; therefore, the compound is highly dissolved in fatty compartments from which it is slowly eliminated over days or weeks, as has been observed for *DDT*

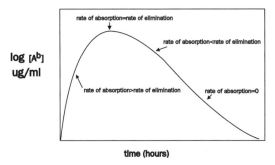

Figure 4
Absorption and elimination of an oral dose.

and *TCDD*. These compounds would exhibit very low bioavailability in terms of the proportion of the dose actually available in the plasma.

Typical clinical drugs are eliminated in just a few hours; however, there is a recent trend for some categories of pharmaceuticals to have slower kinetics. This is due to the targeting of drugs toward membrane bound receptors and the need to increase lipophilicity for effectiveness. In order to accurately assess slow kinetics, it is usually necessary to have very sensitive analytical techniques available so that small concentrations of the drug can be measured in the plasma.

REFERENCES

Joly, J. M. and Brown, T. M., Metabolism of aspirin and procaine in mice pretreated with *O*-4-nitrophenyl methyl(phenyl)phosphinate or *O*-4-nitrophenyl diphenylphosphinate, *Toxicol. Appl. Pharmacol.*, 84, 523, 1989.

Gilman, A. G., Rall, T. W., Nies, A. S., and Taylor, P., *The Pharmacological Basis of Therapeutics*, 8th ed., Pergamon Press, New York, 1990.

Klaassen, C. D. and Rozman, K., Absorption, distribution, and excretion of toxicants, in *Casarett and Doull's Toxicology*, Amdur, M. O., Doull, J., and Klaassen, C. D., Eds., Pergamon Press, New York, 1991, chap. 3.

Shargel, L. and Yu, A. B. C., *Applied Biopharmaceutics and Pharmacokinetics*, 2nd ed., Appleton-Century-Crofts, Norwalk, CT, 1985.

3   BIOTRANSFORMATION

INTRODUCTION

The previous chapter began a discussion of the *toxicokinetic phase*. This phase consists of movement (Greek: *kinesis*) of a poison in the body, including absorption into the circulatory system, distribution among tissues including sites of action, and elimination from the body. This chapter focuses in more detail on the aspect of elimination which involves the loss of the parent drug from the body due to *biotransformation* of the parent drug to *metabolites*. This biotransformation then generally aids in the excretion of the parent drug in urine or feces.

Metabolites are the products of enzyme-catalyzed chemical changes in a drug or toxicant. These products may vary in toxicity and/or therapeutic effect from the parent drug or toxicant. When biotransformation results in a less toxic product, the process is *detoxification*. Some reactions, however, lead to the formation of products which are more toxic than the parent. These reactions are known as *intoxication* or *bioactivation* reactions. In many cases, the parent drug or toxicant is reversibly bound to a protein, or otherwise temporarily sequestered, only to be released again into the blood as the parent compound at a later point.

In general, blood-borne drugs and toxicants are most capable of crossing cell membranes and binding to protein targets if they are *lipophilic*, small, and neutrally charged. Detoxification, then, is most efficient when the parent compound can be altered to a metabolite which is *hydrophilic*, large, and carries a charge. These changes typically occur in two stages. First, in what is often referred to as *Phase I reactions*, the parent compound is typically *hydrolyzed* or *oxidized* (or in some cases, reduced). This leads to formation of a metabolite which is then *conjugated* (bound) to a larger, much more hydrophilic molecule, which often carries a charge. This second conjugation step is often referred to as a *Phase II reaction*. Usually, this stepwise biotransformation is necessary due to the lack in the parent compound of a functional group for easy conjugation.

As an example, carbohydrates are often involved in conjugation reactions. Many carbohydrates are very soluble in water (consider the teaspoons of sucrose which dissolve readily to sweeten your coffee or tea) when a toxicant is conjugated to a carbohydrate, it becomes very water soluble as well. The result is that this product molecule, or *conjugate*, shows little tendency to partition into lipids or membranes, and is instead easily excreted in urine.

A revolution is occurring in toxicology with methods developed in the field of molecular genetics. Enzymes for xenobiotic biotransformation are studied by proteinless sequencing in which the gene is cloned and sequenced, and then the protein sequence is inferred by translating the codons present in the gene sequence. This method is much faster and easier than enzyme purification and protein sequencing methods. Much of the information in this chapter was derived through application of such techniques. Another important contribution of molecular biology is the development of diagnostic tests for genetic deficiencies. Patients with a low level of detoxicative capacity can be identified, and in some cases the deficiency in these "poor metabolizers" has been traced to a specific change in the sequence of a gene.

PRIMARY BIOTRANSFORMATION (PHASE I REACTIONS)

A drug ingested into the body is subject to the same type of biotransformation as a molecule of food. In both cases, the type of reaction depends on the chemistry of the substance, and on whether or not the substance is a substrate for various enzymes which enhance the efficiency of biotransformation. *Hydrolysis* and *oxidation* are two of the most important primary or Phase I reactions of biotransformation.

Hydrolysis

Methoprene, an insecticide used for mosquito and fly control, possesses similar chemistry to a fatty acid alkyl ester (Figure 1). Esters are subject to *hydrolysis* during which they are split with water to yield an acid and an alcohol. (This is the reverse of *esterification* in which an acid and an alcohol react to produce an ester accompanied by water.) Hydrolysis proceeds more rapidly in alkaline conditions because it is actually the hydroxyl ion which attacks an electrophilic carbon in the reaction. When fed to cattle, methoprene does not accumulate because it is hydrolyzed to produce isopropanol and an aliphatic acid metabolite. The acid product is then oxidized to carbon dioxide and water. Drugs such as aspirin, propanidid, and procaine, and pesticides such as malathion, its biotransformation product, malaoxon (Figure 1), and pyrethrins also contain an ester linkage (a *carboxylester*) in the molecule, and can also be hydrolyzed.

At the opposite extreme is the insecticide and fire retardant *mirex*—a carcinogen which is no longer being used. The unusual structure of this insecticide (a cage consisting of only carbon and chlorine, see appendix) renders it practically impervious to biotransformation. Mirex has no ester present; therefore, there is no

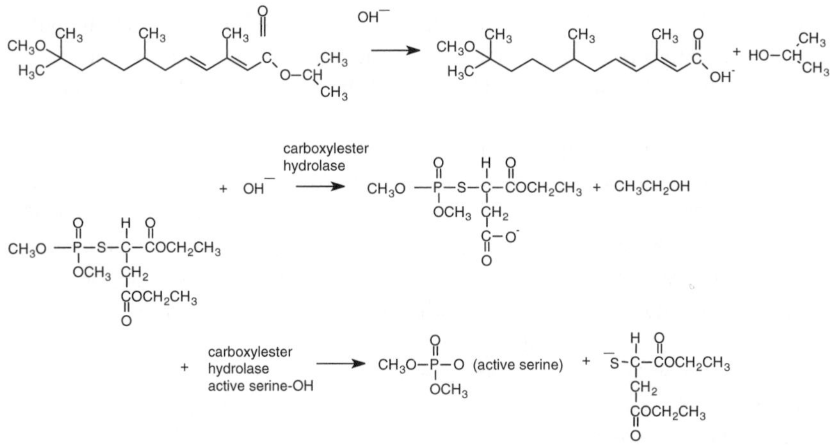

Figure 1 Hydrolysis of methoprene (top) and malathion (bottom).

opportunity for ester hydrolysis. Mirex was found to accumulate in human adipose tissue and in wildlife tissue due to the combination of lipophilicity and very slow biotransformation.

The enzymes which catalyze the hydrolysis reaction are called *hydrolases*. Hydrolases include *amidases* and *peptidases* which are important in the digestion of protein in the diet, and *lipases* which cleave fatty acid esters and glycerides. In addition, *cholinester hydrolases* are active in hydrolysis of choline esters. Among the hydrolases of the liver are several which detoxify important endogenous and xenobiotic carboxylesters. These *carboxylester hydrolases*, known for detoxication of xenobiotics, are likely also to function as lipases in lipid digestion.

Peptidases, carboxylester hydrolases, and cholinester hydrolases are also known as *serine hydrolases* because the catalytic site is a serine residue which reacts with the substrate to form a transiently alkylated enzyme as the ester bond of the substrate is cleaved. Serine hydrolase genes have been cloned and the enzymes have been found to contain highly conserved regions of amino acid sequences, especially a Phe-Gly-Glu-Ser-Ala-Glu sequence which includes the serine at the catalytic site.

In the peptidases chymotrypsin and trypsin, the three dimensional structure of the enzyme is known from *X-ray crystallography*. Serine[195] of the catalytic site is part of a *catalytic triad* of amino acids residues which also includes histidine[57] and aspartic acid.[102] The nucleophilicity of serine[195] is enhanced by charge transfer from aspartic acid[102] to histidine[57] which accepts the proton of the serine hydroxy[195] group as it attacks the substrate. *Site-directed mutagenesis* (the technique of inducing a specific mutation in a gene) consisting of the substitution of asparagine[102] for the aspartic[102] acid destroyed the activity of the enzyme without disturbing the configuration of the triad, demonstrating the importance of the charge transfer phenomenon and the role of the aspartic acid[102] in the activity of serine.[195]

Shape is also important in the active sites of hydrolases. Carboxylesters and amides form a *tetrahedral transition state* when attacked by serine[195] prior to the cleavage of the leaving alcohol or amine. The three dimensional shape of the enzyme forces the substrate into the active site in an orientation which favors formation of the transition state, the conformation from which the reaction can proceed most readily. By favoring this orientation, the enzyme lowers the activation energy required for hydrolysis.

The carboxylester hydrolases are very diverse group, with more than 20 genes in mouse, and multiple genes in rat and in humans. In mouse, there are two clusters of carboxylester hydrolase genes on chromosome 8 and several additional genes on other chromosomes. This characteristic suggests a *multigene family*. The evolution of multigene families may have involved the duplication of genes on a chromosome followed by the divergence of the duplicated genes leading to a cluster of different, but related, genes encoding enzymes of similar function whose activity taken together can catalyze a broad spectrum of reactions.

Cholinester hydrolases are active against *choline esters*; carboxylesters in which the leaving group alcohol is the quaternary amine, *choline*. *Acetyl-cholinesterase* (acetylcholine hydrolase) is a critical enzyme for clearing the neuromuscular synapse of the neurotransmitter, *acetylcholine*. Acetylcholinesterase is the target of poisoning by many organophosphorus and carbamate pesticides. Acetylcholinesterase is present in many tissues, including the erythrocytes, from which its activity can be monitored conveniently. Activity against carboxylester substrates declines as the acyl

---

ACETYLCHOLINESTERASE:
see also:
   Cellular sites of action   *Ch. 4, p. 39*
   Neurotoxicology   *Ch. 9, p. 130*
   Organophosphates *Appendix, p. 242*

---

group is lengthened from acetate. In the serum, *butyrylcholine hydrolase* is a similar enzyme with activity against longer chained acyl esters. There is only one gene each for acetylcholinesterase and butyrylcholinesterase in humans.

Recent X-ray crystallography of acetylcholinesterase from *Torpedo californica* has revealed a gorge extending very deep into the enzyme. At the bottom of the gorge is the active site with serine as part of a catalytic triad composed of glutamic acid,[327] histidine,[440] and serine[200] (similar to the aspartic acid,[102] histidine,[57] and serine[195] triad of chymotrypsin). A pocket at the bottom of the gorge is lined with phenylalanine residues which restrict the acyl group of the substrate to acetate. Sequence comparison indicated that a more spacious pocket is present naturally in butyrylcholinesterase and in lipases which must accept substrates bearing large acyl substituents. It is possible by site-directed mutagenesis to open the acetylcholinesterase active site acyl pocket to introduce very efficient butyryl-cholinesterase activity while retaining acetylcholinesterase activity. This appears to have happened in insecticide resistant acetylcholinesterases of several agricultural pest insects which formerly lacked butyrylcholinesterase activity.

Pesticidal organophosphate esters react rapidly and irreversibly with the active serine of carboxylester hydrolases and peptidases, inhibiting these enzymes. Although this reaction with serine hydrolases is a factor in the detoxication of these potent poisons, the reaction leaves the serine phosphorylated,

MALATHION
see also:
   Organophosphates   Appendix, p. 242

the enzyme activity lost, and thus one mole of serine hydrolase is sacrificed for each mole of organophosphate degraded. *Malathion* is a substrate for carboxylester hydrolases, and in fact is primarily metabolized through hydrolysis of its carboxylester group. The metabolic product of malathion is *malaoxon*, which is a more reactive acetylcholinesterase inhibitor than malathion. Malaoxon possesses both a substrate carboxylester group and an inhibitor phosphorothionate group. Malathion carboxylester hydrolysis proceeds linearly; however, malaoxon carboxylester hydrolysis is progressively inhibited resulting in a progressive decline of hydrolysis. While malaoxon is unusual in serving as both substrate and inhibitor for carboxylester hydrases, the general pathways of intoxicative and detoxicative biotransformation illustrated by malathion apply to most organophosphorothioate pesticides (Figure 2). Toxicity from these compounds depends on the rates of bioactivation vs. detoxification—both of which are affected by factors which alter metabolism.

In mammalian liver and serum, there is a *paraoxonase* which can also catalyze organophosphate hydrolysis (but by an unknown mechanism). Nothing resembling the serine-containing conserved sequence of the serine hydrolases is found in paraoxonase. Thus, this type of enzyme is not likely to possess a serine active site, but perhaps uses a cysteine residue as do *thiol hydrolases* such as

(parent compound) → *detoxication path*
        ↓
intoxication path

P=S → *detoxication*
   ↓
P=O → *detoxication*
   ↓
phosphorylated acetylcholinesterase

malathion → *malathion carboxylic acid*
        ↓
malaoxon → *malathion carboxylic acid*
        ↓
phosphorylated acetylcholinesterase

Figure 2   Pathways of metabolism of organophosphates.

papain. Also, when a number of *chiral* organophosphate inhibitors (those which possess four unlike substituents of phosphorus and therefore exist as either (+) or (−) *enantiomers*) were evaluated as substrates for both types of enzymes, acetyl-cholinesterase and chymotrypsin usually preferred the opposite enantiomer compared to paraoxonase. This suggests that the shape of the active site in paraoxonase is the mirror image of the active sites of acetylcholinesterase and chymotrypsin. Still, acetylcholinesterase and paraoxonase likely have active sites of similar size (but smaller than either the peptidase chymotrypsin or carboxylester hydrolase).

Paraoxonases are common in mammals, but very rare in birds and insects. In humans, there is a polymorphism in the activity of paraoxonase in serum, with a low-activity allele and a high-activity allele. Caucasians have a low-activity allele with a frequency of 50 to 70%, while Africans and Asians have primarily the high activity allele, and South Pacific aboriginal tribes have only the high-activity form.

Oxidation

Oxidation is a second mechanism of primary metabolism by which xenobiotics are detoxified, or sometimes bioactivated to a more toxic product. A wide variety of oxidation reactions are catalyzed by *cytochrome P450* enzymes of various forms in *microsomes* of the *smooth endoplasmic reticulum* of the liver. Also known as monooxygenases, P450 enzymes include a *heme* group in which molecular oxygen is bound to iron. P450 is named for the characteristic peak of light absorbance at 450nm, when *carbon monoxide*, a potent inhibitor, is bound to the reduced enzyme and scanned vs. the reduced enzyme as a reference. This is called the *ferrous-CO 450nm Soret band.*

P450 genes are members of an anciently evolved multigene superfamily in bacteria, plants, and animals. Within a species, there may be members of several gene families for one type of enzyme. For example, there are 36 known families of P450 enzymes based on protein sequence homology, and all mammals studies to date have at least one representative gene from each of 12 different P450 families. While some P450 genes in one family occur in clusters, 15 genes have been mapped to 7 different human chromosomes.

In these P450 families there is a conserved Phe-X-X-Gly-X-X-X-Cys-X-Gly sequence near the cysteine residue which holds the heme molecule in position. Apart from this heme binding site, however, there is a great diversity of sequence, with each P450 family consisting of proteins with >40% sequence homology. Some families have a relatively broad range of substrates which overlap to other families. P450 families are numbered using a somewhat arbitrary system in which some numbers were assigned to preserve continuity in the literature.

Many of the P450 enzymes can undergo the process of *induction*, whereby enzyme activities increase following exposure to substrates. Major inducing agents include phenobarbital, which induces the synthesis of one group of P450 enzymes, and 3-methylcholanthrene (3-MC) and TCDD, which induce the synthesis of a separate group of P450 enzymes. Although the mechanism for phenobarbital induction is not well understood, induction by 3-MC and related compounds has been explained through a series of experiments. Investigations in mice led to the discovery of a soluble protein receptor, or *transcription factor*, called the *Ah receptor*, which was lacking in homozygous mutant *Ah⁻* mice. Mice with the Ah receptor, which has a high affinity for TCDD, were susceptible to poisoning by TCDD; however, *Ah⁻* mice were not responsive. After binding of 3-MC or TCDD to the Ah receptor, the whole complex translocates to the nucleus where interaction with DNA results in transcription of the appropriate P450 genes.

P450 activity can also be inhibited. Inhibitors of protein synthesis can block the induction process, and some compounds can act as specific competitive inhibitors for binding to the P450 enzyme. Examples include carbon monoxide, which competes with oxygen for binding to the heme site, and compounds such as piperonyl butoxide, and a compound called SKF 525-A compete for binding at the substrate binding site.

In P450-catalyzed reactions oxygen is activated by two electrons and then one oxygen atom is inserted into the substrate drug, and the other oxygen atom is reduced to yield water. During these steps P450 must be reduced first, then bind substrate and molecular oxygen to complete the oxidation reaction. Reduction is accomplished by electron transport from *NADPH cytochrome P450 reductase*. Both enzymes are embedded adjacently in the microsomal membrane allowing efficient reduction of P450. Reduced P450 can activate molecular oxygen for substrate oxidation. The general P450-catalyzed oxidation reaction is:

$$\text{substrate(H)} + O_2 + \text{NADPH} + H^+ \; \text{—P450} \rightarrow \text{substrate(OH)} + H_2O + \text{NADP}$$

Common reactions catalyzed by P450 include hydroxylation, dealkylation, and epoxidation. Oxidation reactions change hydrophobic substrate into more polar products, which can then be conjugated and eliminated through excretion in the urine. Oxidative biotransformation via P450 occurs for a great number of hydrophobic substrates. These substrates include endogenous biochemicals such as steroid hormones, fatty acids and retinoids, as well as many important xenobiotics such as drugs, antibiotics, pesticides, industrial solvents, dyes, and petroleum are substrates. Natural toxins from microorganisms and plants can also be substrates of P450.

One major category of oxidation reactions is *aliphatic hydroxylation*. An example of an aliphatic hydroxylation reaction is shown in Figure 3, which shows the P450-mediated hydroxylation of lauric acid. Other substrates for aliphatic hydroxylation include straight-chain alkanes from hexane to hexadecane, cyclohexane, hexobarbital, and prostaglandins. This reaction is among those catalyzed by *CYP4* (cytochrome P450 family 4), a family characterized by its induction by *clofibrate*, an antihyperlipoproteinemic drug used to decrease lipid levels in the blood after surgery to reduce the risk of clotting. A gene cod-

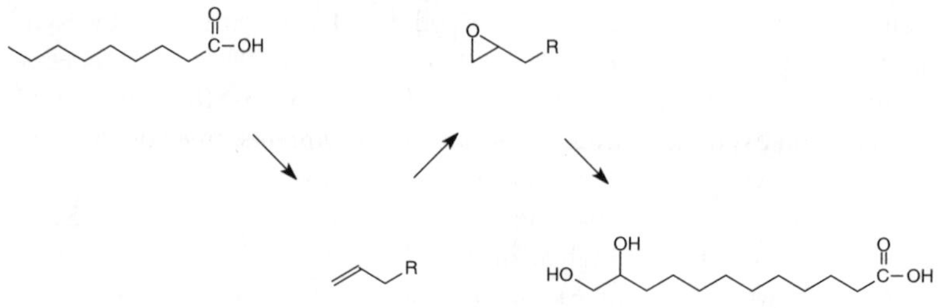

Figure 3   Aliphatic hydroxylation of lauric acid.

ing for one of these proteins was recently found in the cockroach, and shows greater similarity to mammalian CYP4 genes than to several insect genes from other P450 families. This supports the hypothesis that genes for P450 evolved before divergence of the vertebrates and the invertebrates. A unique sequence which serves as a "fingerprint" for proteins from this family is a sequence of 13 consecutive amino acids which are fully conserved within CYP4 but found intact in no other families.

Aliphatic oxidation reactions of steroid hormones are also catalyzed by specific P450 families. The family CYP2A is specific for testosterone 7-α-hydroxylation and is inducible by 3-MC. In the biosynthetic pathway from cholesterol to steroid sex hormones oxidations in positions 17 and 21 (side chain) are catalyzed by families CYP17 and CYP21, and 11-β-hydroxylation is catalyzed by CYP11 (Figure 4).

The antihypertensive *debrisoquin* is hydroxylated by CYP2D, a family which may be involved in biotransformation of many drugs. Metabolic capabilities of this enzyme family can vary from individual to individual, and patients can be characterized as extensive metabolizers or poor metabolizers based on a *polymerase chain reaction* assay of their DNA. Poor metabolizers

---

CARCINOGENESIS
see also:
   Carcinogenesis   *Ch. 5, p. 55*

---

may suffer from deficiency in detoxication of drugs. On the other hand, poor metabolizers among Nigerian cigarette smokers were found to be less susceptible to cancer than extensive metabolizers who smoke, perhaps due to reduced bioactivation of carcinogens in tobacco smoke.

A second type of oxidation is *aromatic hydroxylation*, a characteristic reaction catalyzed by *CYP1* and induced by *TCDD* or *3-MC*. Some aromatic substrates can be hydroxylated by direct insertion of oxygen to produce hydroxylated aromatic rings, such as in the hydroxylation of chlorobenzene to form *ortho-*, *meta-* and *para-*chlorophenols (Figure 5). Others are hydroxylated through initial formation of a transient *epoxide* (arene oxide), which then may undergo hydrolysis to form a more stable metabolite. An example of this is the hydroxylation of

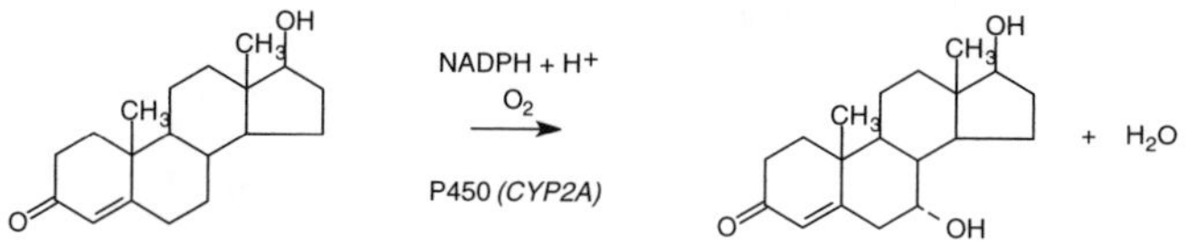

7a-hydroxytestosterone

Figure 4   Aromatic hydroxylation of testosterone.

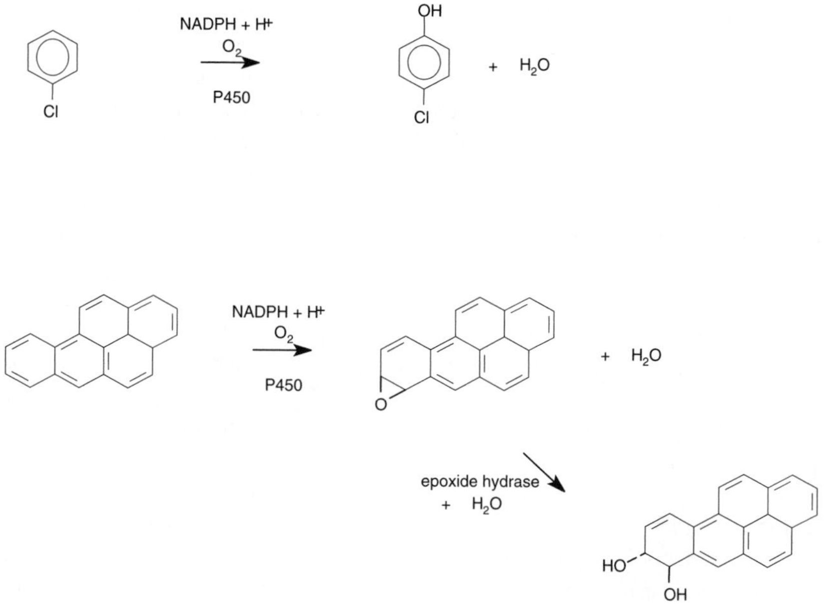

Figure 5   Aromatic hydroxylations of chlorobenzene (top) and benzo[a]pyrene (bottom).

benzo[a]pyrene to form benzo[a]pyrene-7,8-epoxide. This product can then be converted to benzo[a]pyrene-7,8-diol, by addition of water as catalyzed by the enzyme *epoxide hydrolase* (epoxide hydrase) (Figure 5). Aromatic hydroxylation reactions are implicated in bioactivation of carcinogens through formation of reactive epoxide intermediates. For example, benzo[a]pyrene-7,8-diol is a proximate carcinogen which can be further epoxidated to form benzo[a]pyrene-7,8-diol-9,10-epoxide, which is even more reactive with DNA than the parent molecule.

Another common reaction is *alkene oxidation*. One example of alkene oxidation is the epoxidation of the cyclodiene insecticide aldrin, to the 6,7-epoxide product dieldrin (Figure 6). Another cyclodiene, chlordane, is metabolized to heptachlor epoxide. Dieldrin and chlordane were registered for many uses in agricul-

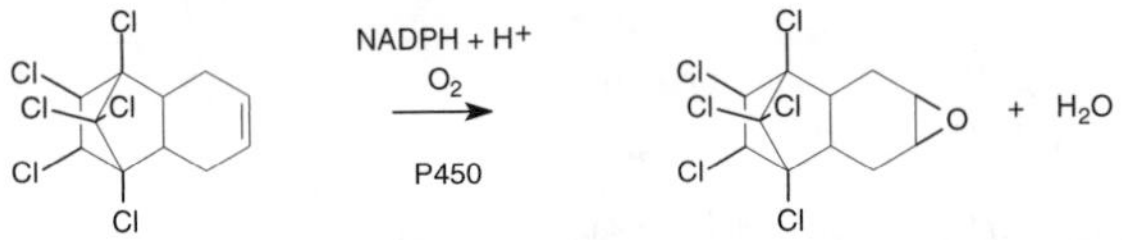

Figure 6 Alkene oxidation of aldrin.

ture, and chlordane was the principal termite proofing agent used over the past 30 years. However, the registrations of these and most other cyclodiene insecticides have been canceled by the EPA due to persistence and suspected carcinogenicity.

An example of an oxidative *O-, S-, or N-dealkylation* is the dealkylation of chlordimeform to form *N*-demethyl chlordimeform which is again *N*-dealkylated to form *N,N*-didemethyl chlordimeform (products which are successively more toxic; Figure 7). These reactions proceed through the formation of reactive oxygen-inserted intermediates which may be carcinogenic. Dialkylnitrosamines may be activated in this fashion. The final products may also be bioactivated as seen for several pesticides including *chlordimeform* and *chlorfenapyl*. Oxidative removal of both methyl groups from chlordimeform gives a more potent activity *in situ* in the firefly, and *piperonyl butoxide*, a P450 inhibitor, blocks the pesticidal activity against cattle ticks. Chlorfenapyl is a new proinsecticide which is 1000-fold less active as an uncoupler of oxidative phosphorylation than is the *N*-dealkylated product. New drugs and pesticides may be designed with these types of bioactivation reactions in mind. A more hydrophobic prodrug could provide efficient transport to the site of action, then be metabolized to an active polar molecule at the site of action.

S or N oxidation, such as the Si oxidation of aldicarb to aldicarb sulfoxide then to aldicarb sulfone (Figure 8), often leads to products that are equal to, or more toxic than, the parent molecules.

Most organophosphorothioate and organophosphorodithioate insecticides are propesticides which are biotransformed to much more toxic and reactive organophosphates through *desulfuration* reactions. For example, malathion-P = S is transformed through the oxidized intermediate [malathion-P-S-O] to form malathion-P = O (Figure 9). The lower toxicity parent compounds are used rather than the metabolites because the metabolites are much too toxic for practical han-

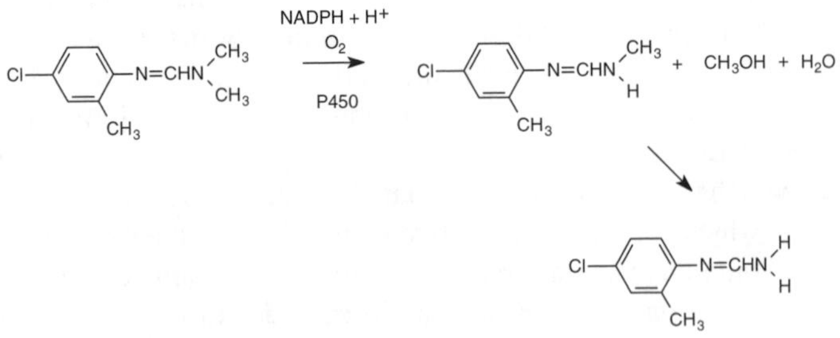

Figure 7 *O, S,* or *N* dealkylation of chlordimeform.

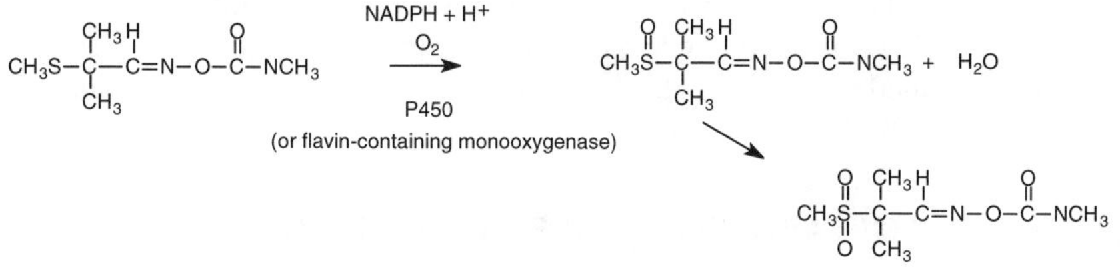

Figure 8   S oxidation of aldicart.

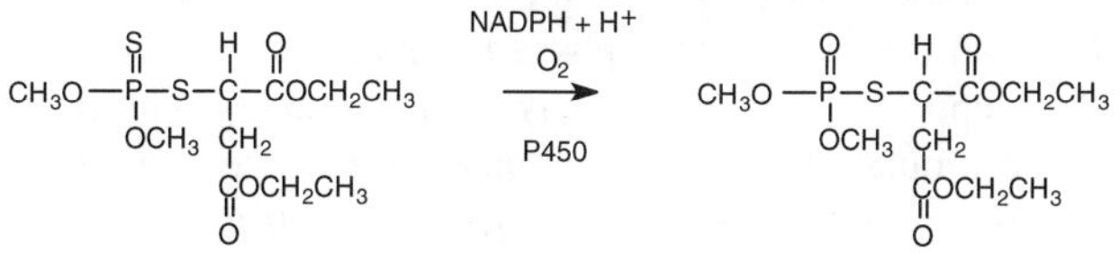

Figure 9   Desulfuration of malathion.

dling and application. About 400 organophosphorothioates active ingredients are applied in agriculture and household pest control and in the control of mosquitoes.

Another class of monooxygenases are the *flavin-containing monooxyge-nases*, which are known for N-oxidation of tertiary amines. These enzymes over-lap with P450 in catalysis of certain biotransformation reactions. They are important in *S*-oxidation reactions and in the desulfuration of phosphonates—those organophosphorus pesticides which possess one phosphorus-to-carbon bond. They are stabilized by the presence of NADPH which, along with molecu-lar oxygen, is required for activity. Like P450, activity is found in liver and kid-ney; however, flavin-containing monooxygenases lack a heme group and are not inhibited by carbon monoxide, nor by piperonyl butoxide. Also, inducers of P450 do not regulate levels of expression of this enzyme.

There are many additional phase I reactions which will not be described in detail. Few other mechanisms are as important for a wide spectrum of xenobiotics as those discussed already. For example, *monoamine oxidase* is a critical enzyme in the brain for *deamination* of neurotransmitters and also for some xenobiotics. It is more significant in pharmacodynamics because it is the target for many enzyme-inhibiting antipsychotic drugs including the original monoamine oxidase inhibitor, *iproniazid*.

Reduction

Some compounds are not oxidized, but are in fact reduced during phase I metabolism. These compounds probably act as electron acceptors, playing the same role as oxygen. In fact, reductions are most likely to occur in environments where oxygen levels are low. Reductions can occur across nitrogen-nitrogen dou-ble bonds (azo reduction) or on nitro (NO_2) groups. Often, the resulting amino compounds can then be oxidized to form toxic metabolites. Halides such as carbon tetrachloride also undergo reduction during their transformation into free radicals. Thus, reduction frequently leads to activation rather than detoxification.

SECONDARY METABOLISM (PHASE II REACTIONS)

Products of phase I may enter a secondary phase of biotransformation in which they are rendered highly polar by conjugation to carbohydrates, amino acids, or small peptides. These products, or conjugates, are excreted from the body more efficiently than the parent or the phase I products. Enzymes which catalyze phase II reactions appear to be coordinately regulated along with phase I so that products do not accumulate when detoxication rates increase. Research in phase II biotransformation is complicated by the need to hydrolyze conjugates with enzymes, such as glucuronidase, peptidase, or sulfatase, in order to recover, identify, and measure the quantity of the phase I product which had been conjugated.

Glucuronidation

Conjugation of phase I products to uridine diphosphoglucuronic acid, a process known as glucuronidation, is catalyzed by the enzyme *UDP-glucuronosyltransferase* found primarily in rough and smooth endoplasmic reticulum. Activity is found in mammalian microsomes from liver, kidney, alimentary tract, and skin. At least eight forms of UDP-glucuronosyltransferases exist in rat liver differing in substrate specificity and inducibility by phenobarbital, 3-MC, and other inducers. Analogous enzymes are encoded by a family of seven or more highly homologous genes in humans. This multigene family displays a diversity of genes within one species and includes individual genes which are conserved among species. These enzyme activities are inducible, some by phenobarbital and some by 3-MC.

Glucuronidation employs the activated nucleoside diphosphate sugar, *uridine diphosphoglucuronic acid* (UDPGA; Figure 10). The first step in synthesis of this cofactor is the reaction of uridine triphosphate (UTP) with glucose-1-phosphate as catalyzed by UDP-glucose pyrophosphorylase. While readily reversible, this reaction is pulled toward synthesis by the rapid hydrolysis of pyrophosphate to orthophosphate catalyzed by pyrophosphatase which leaves only one of the products. The UDP-glucose thus formed is then converted to UDPGA by oxidation of glucosyl C-6 methanol moiety to a carboxyl group.

Glucuronidation is naturally important in the conjugation of *bilirubin*, an endogenous compound produced when heme released from the hemoglobin of dead erythrocytes is oxidized in the spleen. Bilirubin possesses two proprionic acid groups, one of which becomes esterified with glucuronyl from uridine diphosphoglucuronic acid to yield *bilirubin monoglucuronide*. This product is then converted to bilirubin diglucuronide for excretion as the major pigment in

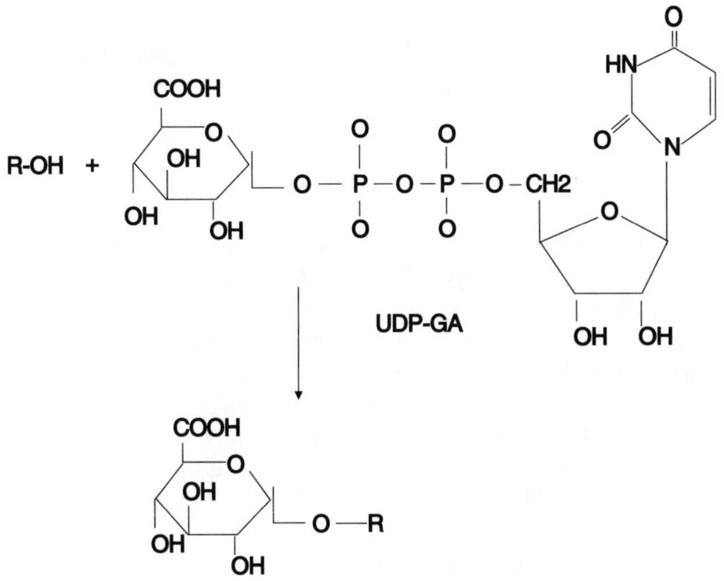

Figure 10 Glucuronidation.

bile (although it appears that the second glucuronidation is accomplished by a different mechanism).

The UDP-glucuronosyltransferase responsible for bilirubin conjugation differs from other, apparently distinct, enzymes which catalyze conjugation of steroids or phenolic xenobiotics. Examples of these reactions include the conjugation of testosterone with UDPGA to form testosterone glucuronide, and the conjugation of 1-naphthol and UDPGA to form naphthyl glucuronide.

In the conjugations described above, the glucuronide conjugation occurs on an oxygen atom resulting in carboxylic acid or ether products. N-, S-, and C-glucuronidation also occurs. While generally detoxicative, formation of N-glucuronides of arylamines and N-hydroxyarylamines may enhance bladder cancer by aiding transport of the carcinogen from the liver to the bladder where the conjugate may undergo acid hydrolysis thus releasing the carcinogen.

In some cases, the parent drug rather than a phase I metabolite may be conjugated directly. Examples of direct glucuronidation include the antihistamine, tripelennamine, which is conjugated to form a quaternary amine N-glucuronide, and the antibiotic, sarafloxacin hydrochloride, for which the most significant biotransformation in chickens and in turkeys is direct glucuronidation.

Glucuronidation is a principal conjugation reaction in most mammals; however, a minor amount of *glucosidation* (conjugation with glucose) has also been detected in mammals. The domestic cat, lion, and lynx fail to produce glucuronides of certain small substrates, but do conjugate bilirubin. On the other hand, glucosidation is the primary conjugation reaction in insects, which coincidentally lack hemoglobin, and in plants. In many insects, phase II reactions are very efficient because certain insecticides are oxidized and excreted primarily as conjugated metabolites.

Glutathione Conjugation

Glutathione is the tripeptide *L*-γ-glutamyl-*L*-cysteinylglycine. This compound has a particularly nucleophilic thiol (sulfhydryl) in the central cysteinyl residue. Glutathione possesses an unusual γ-glutamyl linkage to cysteine; the more common peptide linkage of glutamate is through the carboxyl group bonded to the α-carbon atom. Many tissues are rich in glutathione.

Glutathione can react spontaneously with peroxides and other potentially damaging electrophilic compounds, including certain phase I products of xenobiotics. Some of these reactions are catalytically enhanced by *glutathione transferases*, enzymes with high affinity for lipophilic substances. However, all catalyzed reactions can proceed (although at some slower rate) without the enzyme. These enzymes are coded by a superfamily of at least four multigene families: gst A through gst D. As in the P450 gene superfamily which is known from over 200 sequences, genes of one family can be clustered on a chromosome, or they can be dispersed over several chromosomes. Genes of family gst B are found on three different human chromosomes, while at least six genes of family gst D are tightly clustered on the third chromosome of *Drosophila melanogaster*.

Six forms of glutathione transferases are present in cytosolic fractions of rat and human liver. These forms differ in isoelectric point, but they are similar in size at approximately 23,000 Da per subunit (the enzymes are dimeric). There are also additional glutathione S-transferases found in the microsomes. Besides liver, activity is found in kidney, small intestine, and some other tissues. Activity is found in microorganisms, plants, and throughout the animal kingdom. Site-mutagenesis studies have suggested that a conserved tyrosine residue may be necessary for catalytic activity; however, the precise interactions with substrates has not been determined. Because all reactions occur even without catalysis, it appears that the glutathione sulfhydryl group is the active site and that the enzyme holds it in a position which enhances the nucleophilic attack on the electrophilic substrate, and thus enhances the rate of transition to products.

A wide variety of biotransformation reactions are catalyzed by glutathione transferases. Reduced glutathione is conjugated to a reactive electrophilic carbon, nitrogen, or oxygen atom. One major class of electrophilic compounds which are attacked by glutathione include products of primary detoxication reactions, e.g., arene oxides produced by P450-catalyzed oxidation of xenobiotics discussed in phase I. The resulting glutathione conjugate is metabolized through several reactions converting the glutathione portion to *N*-acetylcysteinyl (*mercapturic acid*), the derivative of the conjugate most commonly detected in urine, and several other products (Figure 11). Glutathione transferases may also play a role in the

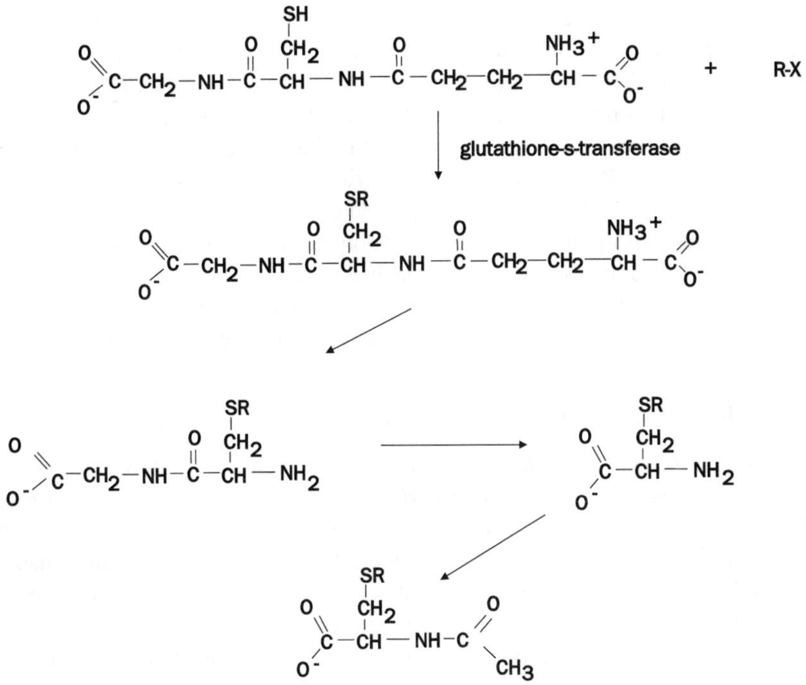

Figure 11 Glutathione conjugation.

detoxication of endogenous lipid and nucleic acid hydroperoxides produced by superoxide radical attack. Linoleic acid hydroperoxide is a good substrate for several glutathione transferases.

The significant role of glutathione transferases in xenobiotic detoxication can be observed in the biotransformation of the common analgesic drug, *acetaminophen* (Tylenol®), which is transformed to *N*-acetyl-*p*-benzoquinonimine, a potential hepatotoxin, in a phase I *N*-oxidation. This reactive product is rapidly conjugated to glutathione in a reaction which is catalyzed readily by glutathione transferases. Depletion of glutathione by acetaminophen overdose negates this detoxication and can lead to liver toxicity or death in extreme cases.

Chemical weed control with *atrazine* in maize is possible because the maize glutathione transferase efficiently detoxifies atrazine. Atrazine is used in greater quantity than any other pesticide in the U.S., primarily for maize. Both reduced glutathione and glutathione *S*-transferase activity are increased in corn and sorghum crops by adding *herbicide safeners* such as dichlormid and flurazole to certain herbicides. These additives increase the margin of safety, or selectivity between killing the competing weed species and the crop plant. The mechanism of increasing glutathione conjugation is unknown, but the enhancement of glutathione *S*-transferase appears to be via induction of transcription from secondary genes.

Glutathione transferases are important in various aspects of cancer research. *Aflatoxin B1* is a mutagen in the Ames test when activated by liver microsomal fraction. The epoxide of aflatoxin B1 formed by P450-catalyzed oxidation can be conjugated with glutathione at a slow rate and induction of higher rates of conjugation decreases the oncogenicity. On the other hand, 1,2-dibromoethane (*ethylene dibromide [EDB]*), a once common agricultural fumigant canceled by the EPA, is biotransformed to a highly carcinogenic glutathione conjugate which acts as a sulfur mustard to alkylate DNA. This activation is probably responsible for the high rate and rapid formation of stomach and nasal carcinoma observed in rats administered 1,2-dibromoethane. In some cases, tumors become resistant to antineoplastic agents due to the high expression of glutathione transferases.

Acetylation and Other Phase II Reactions

Acetylation is an important transformation of arylamines and hydrazines (but not phenols) catalyzed by an *acetyl-CoA-dependent N-acetyltransferase*. Although often detoxicative, acetylation may not lead to a more hydrophilic product, and in some cases, may yield a better substrate for P450 or other phase I enzymes. Common xenobiotic substrates include isoniazid, benzidine, procainamide, and *p*-aminobenzoic acid. This mechanism is greatly reduced in dogs and foxes, and there is a common recessive allele for slow acetylation in humans.

In addition to glucuronidation, glutathione conjugation, and acetylation, many other phase II reactions are known. These include conjugations of phase I products to sulfate, glucose, glycine, and other molecules catalyzed by the respective transferase enzymes.

REFERENCES

Matsumura, F., *Toxicology of Insecticides*, Plenum Press, New York, 1984.

Nebert, D. W. and Gonzalez, F. J., P450 genes: structure, evolution and regulation, *Annu. Rev. Biochem.*, 56, 945, 1987.

Nebert, D. W., and Nelson, D. R., P450 gene nomenclature based on evolution, in *Cytochrome P450*, Waterman, M. R. and Johnson, E. F., Eds., Academic Press, San Diego, CA, 1991, p. 3.

Ravichandran, K. G., Boddupalli, S. S., Hasemann, C. A., Peterson, J. A., and Deisenhofer, J., Crystal structure of hemoprotein domain of P450BM-3, a prototype for microsomal P450s, *Science*, 261, 731, 1993.

Sipes, I. G. and Gandolfi, A. J., Biotransformation of toxicants, in *Casarett and Doull's Toxicology*, Klaassen, C. D., Amdur, M. O., and Doull, J., Eds., Macmillan, New York, 1986, chap. 4.

Sussman, J. L., Harel, M., and Frolow, F., Atomic structure of acetylcholinesterase from *Torpedo californica*: a prototypic acetylcholine-binding protein, *Science*, 253, 872, 1991.

Wislocki, (Reactions catalyzed by P450) in *Enzymatic Basis of Detoxication*, Jacoby, Ed., 1981.

4 CELLULAR SITES OF ACTION

INTRODUCTION

Many toxic substances are known to cause poisoning through a chain of events which begins with action at a very specific target. Often this target is a biological molecule with which the toxicant binds or reacts, such as one or more of the various types of proteins, lipids, and nucleic acids within the cell. Symptoms resulting from exposure to a toxicant may relate directly to this molecular event, or may be complicated by secondary effects (just as symptoms of a disease may be due to physiological imbalances which are secondary to the initial infection). Therefore, identification of the primary site of action requires careful collection and interpretation of biochemical and physiological evidence. For some toxicants, this initial event in poisoning, or "molecular lesion" has been characterized. For many other toxicants, the precise interaction of the toxicant with one or more specific biomolecules has yet to be demonstrated. With the increasingly powerful experimental techniques available, however, it is likely that precise molecular sites of action will be described for many more toxicants in the near future.

This chapter discusses some of the ways in which toxicants are known to interact with biological molecules, as well as some of the techniques used to study these interactions.

INTERACTION OF TOXICANTS WITH PROTEINS

Proteins are composed of a linear chain of amino acids linked together by peptide bonds. The order of the amino acids in a particular protein (known as the protein's *primary structure*) is specified by the sequence of nucleotide codons in a segment of DNA known as a gene. (DNA contains many genes, each one containing the instructions for making one specific amino acid chain.) This DNA nucleotide sequence is transcribed (copied) into messenger RNA, and translated into an amino acid chain on the ribosomes in the cytoplasm of the cell. Portions of the amino acid chain may adopt the form of a helical or pleated sheet (known as *secondary structure*) and these features contribute to the overall general shape (*tertiary structure*) of the protein. Some protein molecules are an aggregation of two or more subunits which may be identical or may be coded for by different genes. The way in which these subunits fit together is called the *quaternary structure* of the protein.

Proteins can play a variety of structural and functional roles within the cell. Tubulin, actin, and other structural proteins comprise the *cytoskeleton* of the cell, providing physical support and also figuring prominently in cell *motility* (movement of a cell or structures within a cell). Some proteins function as *hormones*, carrying messages between cells; others function as the *receptors* on cell surfaces that hormones and other messengers bind to. Proteins also make up the *ion channels* that regulate the flow of ions across cell membranes. *Transport* proteins such as hemoglobin move substances through the bloodstream; other proteins called antibodies defend the body as part of the *immune system*. Finally, protein catalysts called *enzymes* regulate biochemical reactions. Although toxicants can and do interact with all of these types of proteins, this chapter focuses on the effects of toxicants on enzymes, receptors, ion channels, and transport proteins.

Effects of Toxicants on Enzymes

Enzymes are catalysts, meaning that they enhance the rate of various biochemical reactions in the cell. Usually, an enzyme only catalyzes one specific type of reaction. *Substrates* (molecules which participate in the reaction) interact with the *active site* of the enzyme, and are converted to *product*, leaving the enzyme chemically unchanged. Enzyme activity may be modified when binding of the substrate or another molecule to a separate *allosteric site* changes the shape or *conformation* of the enzyme molecule, thus affecting its catalytic ability.

The rate of an enzyme-catalyzed reaction depends primarily on the concentration of the substrate. The greater the substrate concentration, the more enzyme becomes bound to substrate, and the faster the reaction proceeds. Finally, the enzyme becomes *saturated* with substrate, and the velocity approaches a maximum, called the V_{max}. The concentration of substrates at which the rate of reaction is half of the V_{max} is called the *Michaelis constant* (K_m) for that substrate (Figure 1).

Enzyme inhibition is a common molecular mechanism of poisoning. There are two basic types of inhibition, and they can be distinguished on the basis or their different effects on the K_m and V_{max} of the reaction. *Noncompetitive inhibitors* act on an allosteric site and not on the active site. These inhibitors alter the enzyme's catalytic ability in general, reducing the V_{max}; they do not alter the K_m. Inhibitors which compete with the substrate for the active site of an enzyme are called *competitive inhibitors*. Because of their direct competition with the substrate, competitive inhibitors increase the K_m, but their effects can be overcome with large excesses of substrate, and the V_{max} is unaffected. Some competitive inhibitors compete with substrate for binding, but then form a relatively perma-

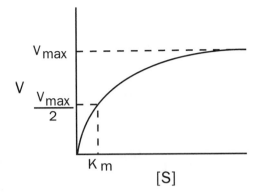

Figure 1
Enzyme kinetics. This figure shows the relationship between K_m and V_{max}.

nent covalent bond with an amino acid at the active site of the enzyme. Because of the permanence of the reaction, this effect is not overcome by excess substrate.

One example of an enzyme as a target for toxicants is the inhibi-tion of the enzyme *acetylcholinesterase* by *organophos- phorus insecticides*. Acetyl-cholinesterase is an enzyme that is important in the passage of impulses between neurons. Communication between neurons is performed by a group of molecules called neurotransmitters, which are released from one neuron, then diffuse across a synaptic gap where they bind to *receptors* on the membrane of the adjoin-ing neuron. Once this process is complete, the synaptic gap must be cleared of neurotransmitters in order to be ready for the next sig-nal. While some neurotransmit-ters are reabsorbed by the releasing neuron, others are bro-ken down by enzymes. Acetylcholinesterase is one such enzyme, clearing the synaptic gap by breaking down the neuro-transmitter acetylcholine.

ACETYLCHOLINESTERASE
see also:
Biotransformation   *Ch. 3, p. 24*
Neurotoxicology   *Ch. 9, p. 130*
Organophosphates   *Appendix, p. 242*

ORGANOPHOSPHATES
see also:
Neurotoxicology   *Ch. 9, pp. 130, 137*
Water pollution   *Ch. 15, p. 217*
Organophosphates   *Appendix, p. 242*

Acetylcholinesterase catalyzes the *hydrolysis* (splitting through the addition of water) of acetylcholine to form choline and acetate. During the catalytic process, an acetyl group ($COCH_3$) from acetylcholine becomes covalently bound to a serine (an amino acid) in the active site of the enzyme (a process called *acetylation*), and a choline molecule is released. Then, because the covalent bond between the enzyme and the acetyl group is not very stable, the acetate is rapidly released. The process is shown in Figure 2. Inhibition involves a similar reaction between the enzyme and the organophosphorus inhibitor at the active site: a

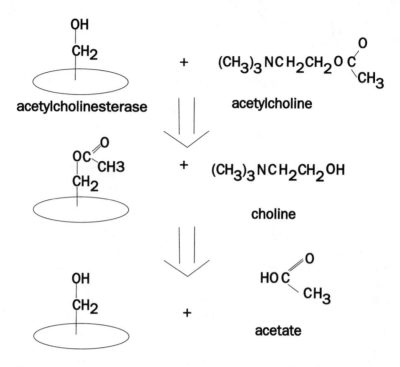

Figure 2   The hydrolysis of acetylcholine by the enzyme acetylcholinesterase.

covalent bond forms, and the serine residue (which normally becomes acety-lated) becomes *phosphorylated* instead (Figure 3). Hydrolysis occurs and part of the inhibitor molecule is released, but the covalent bond formed between the phosphate group and the enzyme is quite stable and may last for at least several hours.

Although based on the time scale of a cell, this inhibition is virtually an *irreversible* process; recovery of the enzyme can occur, however, with the rate of recovery of the phosphorylated enzyme depending on the specific inhibitor. Most commercial organophosphorus insecticides produce a phosphorylated enzyme that takes several hours to recover half its activity. However, inhibition by other insecticides results in a phosphorylated enzyme with a half life of several days. With some insecticides, the phosphorylated enzyme may undergo "*aging,*" during which a chemical change to the phosphoryl group occurs (Figure 4). Aged, phos-phorylated enzyme does not reactivate at all. *Phosphinate inhibitors* are also used, and produce a phosphinylated acetylcholinesterase which does not "age," so that recovery is possible.

Because of the long recovery time, exposure to organophosphorus insecti-cides leads to accumulation of phosphorylated enzyme and thus a decline in active

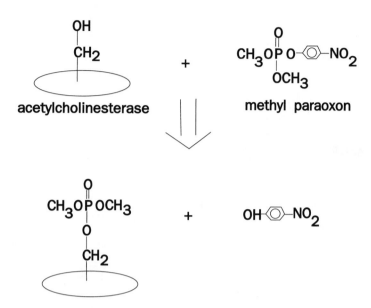

Figure 3   The phosphorylation of the enzyme acetylcholinesterase by the organophosphate insecticide methyl paraoxon.

enzyme levels. The potency of inhibitors can be compared by measuring the rate at which enzyme activity declines. Symptoms of inhibition result when about 60 to 70% of the enzyme is phosphorylated. They are related to an excess of acetylcholine and resulting overstimulation at synapses (1) between nerve and voluntary muscle, (2) in the central nervous system, and (3) in the parasympathetic branch of the autonomic nervous system. These symptoms in humans include constriction of the pupil, slowing of heart rate, excessive salivation, and muscle contraction. The cause of death in poisoning by organophosphorus insecticides is usually asphyxiation caused either by malfunctioning of the diaphragm and the related muscles involved in breathing, or failure of the respiratory center in the brain which controls this process.

Antidotes for organophosphorus toxicants include *2-PAM* which is a base used to promote recovery of phosphorylated acetylcholinesterase. Generally, 2-PAM is used in conjunction with *atropine* which acts as an *antagonist* (blocker) at acetylcholine receptors to counteract the overstimulation from acetylcholine. Poisoning is also treated by providing artificial respiration and general life support.

Other potential targets for toxicants are the various *mitochondrial enzymes*. Mitochondria (Figure 5) are cellular organelles that extract usable energy from glucose and other molecules and transfer it to the high-energy molecule ATP. This process begins with the metabolic pathways of glycolysis and the citric acid

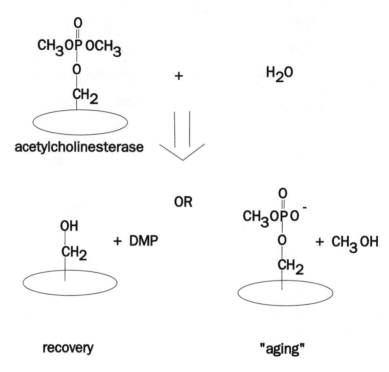

Figure 4   The recovery and "aging" of phosphorylated acetylcholinesterase.

cycle, where glucose is broken down, leading to the reduction of (addition of electrons to) electron acceptor molecules such as NAD^+ or FAD^+. The electrons
gained by these molecules are then transferred to a series of enzyme complexes
and electron carriers called the *respiratory chain*, located within the mitochondrial inner membrane. According to the *chemiosmotic hypothesis*, electrons are
passed down from one member of the chain to the next, until they are eventually
donated to oxygen at the end of the line. As electrons are transported along the
chain, protons are picked up from inside the mitochondrion and carried across the
inner membrane to the space between the inner and outer membranes. Because
the mitochondrial membrane is not very permeable to protons, a concentration
gradient develops that tends to push protons back across the membrane through
protein channels that are part of another enzyme called a Mg^{++} ATPase. The
movement of a pair of protons through the channel drives the synthesis of a molecule of ATP (Figure 6).

    There are several mitochondrial enzymes for which the effects of inhibition by
various toxicants are well documented. One of the most notorious toxic chemicals,
cyanide, blocks electron transport by inhibiting the enzyme complex cytochrome

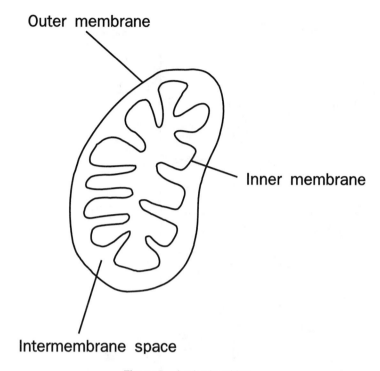

Outer membrane

Inner membrane

Intermembrane space

Figure 5 A mitochondrion.

oxidase, a member of the electron transport chain. Other toxicants, including the pesticide *rotenone*, the barbiturate *amytal*, and the antibiotic *antimycin A* inhibit other enzymes complexes in the chain. When the flow of electrons is blocked by any of these *transport inhibitors*, the final transfer of electrons to an oxygen molecule does not occur. This effect is measurable in the laboratory as a decrease in mitochondrial oxygen uptake. In addition, because the proton gradient does not develop properly, there is a reduction in ATP production (also measurable). Another mitochondrial enzyme which has been shown to be affected by toxicants is the Mg^{++} ATPase. *ATPase inhibitors* such as *oligomycin* inhibit this enzyme, thus blocking the formation of ATP. Inhibition of the ATPase also prevents the discharge of the proton gradient, and because the resulting pressure opposes further proton pumping, electron transport and thus oxygen uptake is also reduced.

A third class of toxicants which acts on mitochondria are known as *uncouplers*. As their name suggests, these toxicants uncouple the two processes of electron transport and ATPase production. The result is a stimulation of electron transport (again, measured by oxygen uptake) along with a reduction in ATP production. There are many different uncouplers, and the mechanism of action of many is not completely clear. Most uncouplers probably interact with membrane proteins or lipids to alter permeability of the membrane to protons, thus interfering with the maintenance of the proton gradient. The oldest synthetic organic

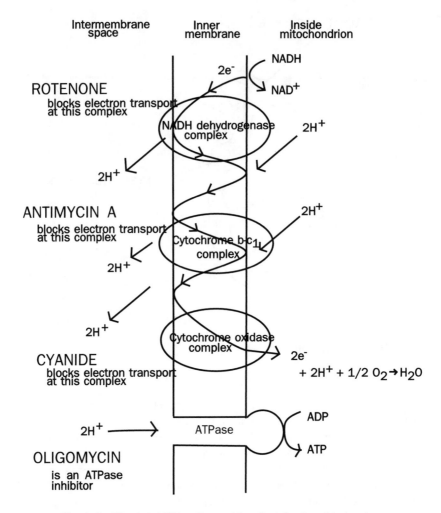

Figure 6   Mitochondrial function and the sites of action of toxicants.

insecticide, dinitro orthocresol (DNOC) is an uncoupler and was once used as a drug to enhance weight loss, because uncoupling allows food to be oxidized without producing ATP. This target has been rediscovered recently with the development of a new insecticide chlorfenapyr (American Cyanamid).

Effects of Toxicants on Receptors and Ion Channels

Receptors are proteins which respond to the binding of a signal molecule generally referred to as a *ligand*. Receptors may be found in membranes, as transmembrane channels, or in the cytoplasm. Ligands may be hormones, neurotransmitters, other internal signaling molecules, or *xenobiotics* (compounds foreign to the body). Generally, binding of ligands to receptors is quite specific, in that only a limited number of ligands (which are generally closely related structurally) will bind to a given receptor. Receptors form a complex with a ligand with kinetics that are similar to the formation of an enzyme-substrate complex. Experimentally, a specific receptor can be detected using a ligand which has been labeled with a radioactive element such as tritium. First, the amount of labeled ligand bound to all protein (including both specific binding to the receptor and nonspecific binding to other molecules in the cell) is measured. Then, the experiment is repeated, but this time with a 100-fold excess of nonlabeled ligand added, also. The idea is that the nonlabeled ligand will bind to the specific receptor, a saturable process, leaving only the nonspecific binding sites for the labeled ligand. When this difference between total and nonspecific binding is measured over a series of labeled ligand concentrations, the binding of ligand to the specific receptor can be estimated.

The protein structures of several receptors have been inferred from the nucleotide sequences of the genes which encode them. Such new techniques in molecular genetics have the potential to revolutionize the understanding of toxicology on the cellular level by allowing for detailed analysis of many proteins which occur at concentrations far too low for conventional purification. First, messenger RNA is extracted from an organism known to produce the protein of interest (the receptor) in relative abundance. The mRNA is then partially purified by chromatography and used as a template for preparing complementary DNA by *reverse transcription*. This process is catalyzed by the enzyme reverse transcriptase (as found in RNA viruses). The resulting complementary DNA can be cut into pieces by enzymes called restriction endonucleases, and the pieces inserted into host bacteria using *vectors* such as bacterial plasmids or viruses which infect bacteria. The bacterial cells then are grown into colonies, with the bacteria in each colony containing a fragment of the DNA of interest.

If a part of the gene sequence is known or can be inferred from a known sequence of amino acids in the protein, then a radioactively labeled probe can be synthesized and used to identify the colonies containing the gene of interest. If the gene sequence is not known, then identification of the proper colonies must be made by testing for the characteristic activity of the protein of interest, e.g., by transcribing mRNA and injecting it into *Xenopus* oocytes, or by immunoassay for the protein (if an antibody for that protein is available). Once the proper piece of DNA is identified, its nucleotide sequence can be determined. To confirm that the right DNA was identified, the cloned DNA can be matched up with mRNA or DNA from the original organism through a technique called hybridization. Once several sequences are known, PCR techniques can be applied to obtain sequences from additional species without further gene cloning.

In contrast to enzymes, receptor proteins do not catalyze chemical reactions; however, binding of ligand to a receptor may result in profound changes such as the opening of an ion channel through a membrane, activation of enzymes through the actions of second messengers, or the triggering of transcription of a gene. One example of interaction of a ligand with a receptor to trigger transcription is the induction of cytochrome P450 by xenobiotics.

P450
see also:
  Biotransformation   ***Ch. 3, p. 26***

The *cytochrome P450-dependent monooxygenases* are a large group of enzymes important in the metabolism and detoxification or activation of many xenobiotic compounds. Levels of the various forms of P450 are responsive to the concentrations of xenobiotics in the body: presence of certain xenobiotics can trigger an increase in synthesis of P450 enzymes, a process called *induction* that is mediated by receptor binding. One chemical with the ability to induce one form of P450 (P450I) synthesis is *dioxin* (TCDD). TCDD enters liver cells (where most xenobiotic metabolism occurs) and binds to a receptor in the cytoplasm. The receptor-ligand complex then moves into the nucleus, where it interacts with the DNA to initiate the transcription of several genes including the gene which encodes the specific enzyme which metabolizes TCDD. Many other xenobiotics with similar chemical structures to TCDD also appear to bind to this cytosolic receptor, and also initiate synthesis of the enzyme. Inducers of other forms of P450 include phenobarbital, ethanol, and other compounds. Inhibitors of P450 include carbon monoxide and piperonyl butoxide.

Several neurotransmitter receptors are actually ligand-activated transmembrane ion channels. These include the *γ-aminobutyric acid (GABA) receptor* and the *acetylcholine receptor* (Figure 7). These neuroreceptors incorporate ion channels which are opened in response to binding by neurotransmitters. GABA receptors incorporate a chloride ion channel and are composed of primary α, β, and Δ subunits. Acetylcholine receptors

---

NEUROTRANSMITTER RECEPTORS
see also:
  Neurotoxicology   ***Ch. 9, p. 125***

---

are more complex with four different genes encoding protein subunits. The α subunit, which binds the neurotransmitter, occurs twice in the molecule along with one of each of the β, γ, and Δ subunits, arranged in a rosette which has been observed by electron microscopy. A small portion of the Δ subunit determines ionic conductance characteristics, as was proved by elegant experiments in which chimeric bovine and *Torpedo* genes were expressed in *Xenopus* oocytes.

The presence of a particular receptor determines the nature of the synapse. When acetylcholine receptors are present in the postsynaptic membrane, the synapse is termed *cholinergic* because it will respond to acetylcholine; *adrenergic* synapses have receptors which respond to norepinephrine; *GABAergic* synapses contain receptors which respond to GABA; and so on for the many different neurotransmitter substances which exist in the nervous system.

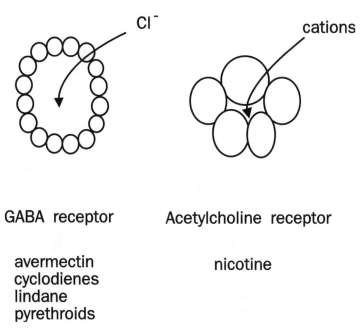

GABA receptor   Acetylcholine receptor

avermectin   nicotine
cyclodienes
lindane
pyrethroids

Figure 7   The GABA and the acetylcholine receptors of respective toxicants.

Receptor classes can be further subdivided by their responses to ligands other than the endogenous neurotransmitter. Ligands which mimic the action of the natural neurotransmitter are known as *agonists*; they bind to the receptor in its active state and elicit a response. *Nicotine* is an agonist of the cholinergic receptors found on skeletal muscle (Type I receptors) among other sites, but is inactive on cholinergic receptors from the parasympathetic nervous system (Type II receptors). Conversely, *muscarine* toxin from the fly agaric mushroom, *Amanita muscaria*, is only agonistic to Type II receptors. These subsets of receptors are also referred to as *nicotinic* or *muscarinic*, respectively.

Antagonists are ligands which bind to the receptor site but do not produce a response. They can negate the action of neurotransmitter or agonist. This can be very useful as in the case of *atropine*, previously discussed as a cholinergic blocker. *Curare*, the muscle relaxant and Amazonian hunter's arrow-tip poison, is an antagonist of Type I cholinergic receptors.

Many ligand-receptor systems also have "second messenger" systems which link the signal produced by binding of the ligand to the receptor with functional changes within the cell. Often, binding activates the enzyme adenyl cyclase, which catalyzes the conversion of ATP into cyclic AMP. Cyclic AMP is then involved in activation of a group of enzymes called protein kinases, which catalyze the phosphorylation of other proteins, leading to changes in cell function. Alternatively, increases in intracellular calcium levels or increased movement of calcium across membranes can also initiate protein phosphorylation. Second mes-

senger systems can also be targets for toxicants. There is some evidence that interference with calcium metabolism, for example, may be a factor in the mechanisms
by which some chemicals produce cell death. Other studies, however, point to
abnormal increases in calcium levels in dying cells as a result rather than as the
cause of cellular injury.

Effects of Toxicants on Voltage-Activated Ion Channels

Another category of transmembrane ion channels includes those which
respond to local voltage change in charged membranes such as the nerve axon.
The passage of an impulse
through the nerve axon is an

ACTION POTENTIAL
see also:
Neurotoxicology   *Ch. 9, p. 121*

electrical phenomenon in that the
impulse is actually a wave of
ionic *depolarization*. Because
neurons are polarized with a negative internal charge, the opening
of sodium ion channels has a depolarizing effect as positive ions flow inward with
the sodium gradient. Once initiated, this depolarization passes completely down
the axon in a wave known as the *action potential*. The action potential requires no
energy; however, once completed, ATP is used to drive ion pumps to restore the
resting gradients.

Upon reaching the presynaptic membrane, the electrical impulse must be
converted into a chemical signal for transmission of the signal to another cell.
First, voltage-activated calcium channels open and calcium flows into the cells
due to a very strong concentration gradient. The change in intracellular calcium
concentration then leads to the release of neurotransmitter.

Both sodium ion channels and potassium ion channels have been described
by cloning and sequencing of the genes which encode them. In the process of
cloning genes for channels, the expression of activity can be observed by injecting messenger RNA into *Xenopus* oocytes which then produce the protein and
incorporate the channels into the oocyte membrane. Voltage stimulus results in
channel opening.

Voltage-activated sodium channels are the molecular site of action of
tetrodotoxin, (TTX) an alkaloid found in skin and gonads of the globe fish,
Spheroides rubripes, and in cer-
tain newts and frogs. Saxitoxin,

TTX, STX
see also:
Cardiovascular
*   toxicology*   *Ch. 8, p.106*
Neurotoxicology   *Chp. 9, p. 123*
TTX, STX   *Appendix, p. 246*

from   the   dinoflagellates
Gonyaulax catenella and *G.
tamatensis* (of poisonous red
tide), also acts specifically on the
sodium ion channel. Both toxins
block the sodium channel and are
among the most toxic natural

occurring chemicals known, with median lethal doses in mice of approximately 10 μg/kg by intraperitoneal injection. Batrachitoxin, on the other hand, increases permeability to sodium. It appears that poisoning of only a small percentage of sodium ion channels can be lethal. This is due to the necessity of maintaining a resting potential which is more negative than the threshold for the action potential. Leakage of sodium ions through a few poisoned channels results in a resting potential which is too close to the threshold, causing hyperexcitability of the neuron.

Effects of Toxicants on Transport Proteins

While there are several different proteins that function in transport, probably the most well known is *hemoglobin*, an oxygen-carrying molecule found in red blood cells. In vertebrates, the hemoglobin molecule is made up of four amino acid chains, with each chain possessing an iron-containing structure called a heme group which is capable of carrying a molecule of oxygen. The binding of oxygen to the heme group of one of the amino acid chains alters the conformation of the remaining chains to make oxygen binding easier. Likewise, the release of oxygen by one heme group produces a conformational change that encourages oxygen release by the other heme groups as well. The net result is that hemoglobin loads oxygen easily in areas rich in oxygen and unloads it promptly in areas low in oxygen. Around 98% of the oxygen in the bloodstream is carried by hemoglobin; the remaining 2% is dissolved in the blood plasma.

Carbon monoxide (CO) is a toxicant which interferes with the functioning of hemoglobin by competing with oxygen for binding to the heme groups. In humans, hemoglobin has a much higher affinity for carbon monoxide than for oxygen (by a factor of 200) so even very small amounts of carbon monoxide can effectively block oxygen binding. Carbon monoxide poisoning is particularly insidious because the potential compensatory responses to oxygen deprivation are not trig-

CARBON MONOXIDE
see also:
   Cardiovascular
     toxicology   *Ch. 8, pp. 110, 114*
   Air pollution   *Ch. 14, p. 202*
   Carbon monoxide   *Appendix, p. 236*

gered by reduction in oxygen binding by hemoglobin, but only by changes in dissolved oxygen levels (which are affected little if at all by moderate levels of carbon monoxide). Thus, in carbon monoxide poisoning there is no sensation of struggling for breath, but just gradual loss of consciousness. Poisoning is treated with oxygen, often with a little carbon dioxide added to stimulate breathing. Under normal circumstances, less than 1% of a person's circulating hemoglobin carries carbon monoxide; for smokers, however, the figure is closer to 5 to 10% because of exposure to the carbon monoxide given off in cigarette smoke.

Another alteration which can prevent hemoglobin from carrying oxygen is the oxidation of the heme iron from the ferrous (Fe^{+2}) to the ferric (Fe^{+3}) state. A hemoglobin molecule with these oxidized heme irons is called *methemoglobin*. A small percentage of circulating hemoglobin exists normally in this state; however, exposure to certain chemicals can dramatically increase methemoglobin levels leading to a condition called *methemoglobinemia*. One such group of chemicals are the *nitrates*. These highly water-soluble compounds found in sewage wastes and fertilizers are frequent groundwater pollutants. They are also used in the processing and preservation of meats. Nitrates are converted in the gastrointestinal system to *nitrites* which then oxidize heme iron to produce methemoglobin.

Methemoglobinemia is relatively rare in adults, because of the existence of a biochemical system that can reduce the oxidized heme iron, converting methemoglobin back to hemoglobin. Infants, however, are deficient in this enzyme, a factor which puts them at special risk. Most cases of methemoglobinemia occur in infants in rural areas where nitrate-contaminated well water is used to prepare formula. Affected babies literally turn blue, but termination of exposure and prompt medical attention usually leads to recovery. One possible treatment for methemoglobinemia is administration of the compound methylene blue, which stimulates reduction of the oxidized heme iron.

Interestingly enough, there is one case in which formation of methemoglobin is deliberately induced, and that is the treatment of cyanide poisoning. Nitrites are administered in order to produce moderate levels of methemoglobin to which cyanide binds to with an even higher affinity than it does for cytochrome oxidase. Administered along with the nitrites is a compound called sodium thiosulfate which converts the cyanide in the bloodstream to thiocyanate (which can then be excreted).

EFFECTS OF TOXICANTS ON LIPIDS

Lipids, of course, play a major role in the structure and function of cell membranes. Cell membranes are composed of a *phospholipid bilayer* (Figure 8) with an internal hydrophobic region consisting of the hydrocarbon "tails" and an external hydrophilic region made up by the phosphate "heads" of the phospholipids. Certain proteins, including receptors and ion channels, have a tertiary structure with strongly hydrophobic regions, allowing them to be imbedded in the membrane. Membranes are *dynamic*, having fluidity as well as constant turnover with incorporation of newly synthesized components.

Highly lipophilic substances may dissolve readily into membranes because they reach much higher equilibrium concentrations in lipid than in the blood. *Organic solvents* and *anesthetic gases* are among the substances with narcotic

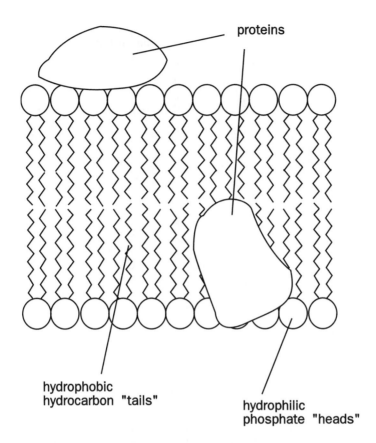

Figure 8   The phospholipid bilayer as found in membranes.

activity which is correlated to lipid solubility. These compounds may dissolve in membranes of the central nervous system, the heart, and other organs, exerting their toxic effects through alteration of membrane structure and function. For example, there is evidence that high concentrations of anesthetics increase lipid fluidity of membranes; however, this effect is not observed at normal anesthetic concentrations.

ORGANIC SOLVENTS
see also:
  Neurotoxicology   *Ch. 9, p. 143*

The fatty acid chains of many membrane phospholipids are unsaturated (contain double bonds). These unsaturated fatty acids are susceptible to damage through a process called *lipid peroxidation*. In lipid peroxidation, free radicals (molecules with unpaired electrons) formed from halogenated hydrocarbons and other xenobiotics attack fatty acids, removing hydrogen atoms and converting the fatty acids into free radicals themselves. These fatty acid free radicals then react with oxygen to

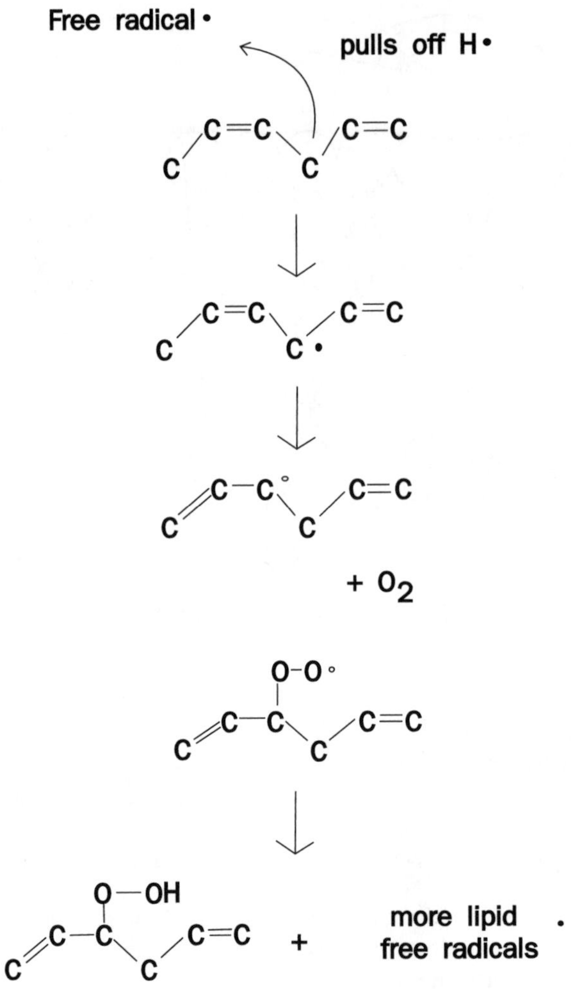

Figure 9 The steps involved in lipid peroxidation.

form additional free radicals and unstable peroxides (which can also break down, yielding even more free radicals). Thus, the process spreads, which can lead to structural and functional damage not only to the plasma membrane, but also to the membranes of cellular organelles such as the endoplasmic reticulum (Figure 9).

EFFECTS OF TOXICANTS ON NUCLEIC ACIDS

DNA is built of units called *nucleotides*, each of which consists of a base (adenine, guanine, cytosine, or thymine), a phosphate, and a deoxyribose sugar. Nucleotides can be linked together through covalent bonds between the phosphate

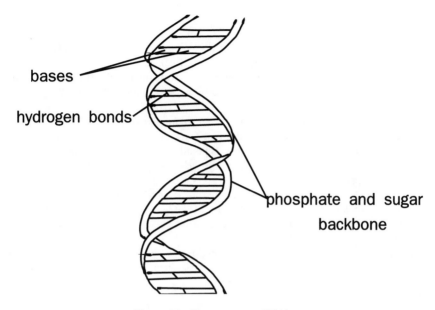

Figure 10   The structure of DNA.

of one nucleotide and the sugar of the next. The DNA molecule itself consists of two *complementary* chains of nucleotides, meaning that each nucleotide in one chain is paired opposite a specific partner in the other chain. A nucleotide containing the base cytosine will always pair with a nucleotide containing the base guanine. Likewise, a nucleotide containing adenine will always pair with a nucleotide containing thymine. The two chains are held together by hydrogen bonds which form between the pairs, and twist together in a form called a double helix (Figure 10).

The toxicants that interact with and produce changes in cellular DNA are described by the general term *mutagens*. Most mutagens interact with the base portions of nucleotides. Some may delete portions of bases,

MUTAGENESIS
see also:
   Carcinogenesis   *Ch. 5, p. 55*

such as nitrous acid which can remove an amine group from adenine or cytosine (a process called *deamination*). Other compounds (mustard gas, for example) act as *alkylating agents*, adding alkyl groups to bases, while still others *replace* nucleotides which they closely resemble. Also, exposure to ultraviolet light and ionizing radiation can cause *cross-linking* between DNA bases. Enzyme systems exist which can deal with such damage, repairing or removing and replacing damaged nucleotides. Unrepaired damage, however, can lead to mutagenicity or carcinogenicity due to misreading or incorrect replication of DNA during cell division. These topics will be discussed in more detail in Chapter 5.

REFERENCES

Grosch, D. S., Genetic poisons, in *Introduction to Biochemical Toxicology*, Hodgson, E. and Guthrie, F. E., Eds., Elsevier, New York, 1980, chap. 14.

Herman, B., Gores, G. J., Nieminen, A.-L., Kawanishi, T., Harman, A., and Lemasters, J. J., Calcium and pH in anoxic and toxic injury, *CRC Crit. Rev. Toxicol.*, 21, 127, 1990.

Main, A. R., Cholinesterase inhibitors, in *Introduction to Biochemical Toxicology*, Hodgson, E. and Guthrie, F. E., Eds., Elsevier, New York, 1980, chap. 11.

Moreland, D. E., Effects of toxicants on oxidative and photophosphorylation, in *Introduction to Biochemical Toxicology*, Hodgson, E. and Guthrie, F. E., Eds., Elsevier, New York, 1980, chap. 13.

Murphy, S. D., Toxic effects of pesticides, in *Casarett and Doull's Toxicology*, Klaassen, C. D., Amdur, M. O., and Doull, J., Eds., Macmillan, New York, 1986, chap. 18.

Rasmussen, H., The cycling of calcium as an intracellular messenger, *Sci. Am.*, October 1989, 66.

Smith, R. P., Toxic responses of the blood, in *Casarett and Doull's Toxicology*. Klaassen, C. D., Amdur, M. O., and Doull, J., Eds., Macmillan, New York, 1986, chap. 8.

5   CARCINOGENESIS

CARCINOGENESIS AND CANCER

Carcinogenesis is the process by which *cancer* develops in the body. Cancer is not a single disease, but rather a general term referring to many kinds of malignant growths which invade adjoining tissue and sometimes spread to distant tissues. *Carcinomas* are cancers of epithelial tissue, while *sarcomas* are cancers of supporting tissues (such as connective or muscle tissues). The most common forms of cancer are carcinomas found in skin, large intestine, bronchi, stomach, prostate gland (in males), breast (usually in females), and cervix in females.

Most current theories describe carcinogenesis as a multistep process, involving three phases beginning with change in one cell and building through an accumulation of factors to the malignant tumor. These three phases are called initiation, promotion, and progression.

Initiation is initial damage to DNA, which may be chemically induced. The initiated cell is considered to be *transformed* into a *neoplastic* cell, but remains latent until affected by promoting agents. *Promotion* is the second phase of the process during which further cellular changes lead to the development of a tumor from the initial neoplastic cell. This stage may be affected by the action of chemical promoters which stimulate cell division to produce clonal proliferation. The importance of promotion in the process of carcinogenesis should not be ignored, and in fact it has been argued that carcinogens requiring very high doses might act through cell damage and the consequential mitogenesis (cell proliferation during the repair process) rather than through any specific mechanism.

The third stage of carcinogenesis is *progression*, during which a tumor becomes malignant. *Benign* tumors are encapsulated, slowly growing, noninvasive and can be controlled by excision; *malignant* tumors are nonencapsulated, rapidly growing, invasive, disseminating, and recalcitrant to treatment. The progression to malignancy is characterized by the aggressive nature of the cells which can attach and penetrate membranes to invade new tissue. *Metastasis* is the process by which a malignant tumor invades and disseminates to other tissues.

Staging is a method for describing the status of a cancer for diagnosis and management. The general classification of each case into stages I to IV is based on scoring system known as TNM, development of the tumor (T), involvement of lymph nodes (N) in the region of the tumor, and degree of metastases (M). For example, the tumor is categorized from T0 (no evidence of a tumor) to T4 (a massive lesion with extensive invasion into adjacent tissues). A combination of clinical, radiographic, surgical, and pathological techniques are used to determine TNM scores. Staging is performed in diagnosis and periodically throughout treatment to evaluate management and remediation of the disease.

CHEMICAL CARCINOGENS

Carcinogens which have the ability to bind to and alter the structure of DNA are called *genetic* carcinogens, while carcinogens which bind to and affect other cellular targets are called *epigenetic* carcinogens. Some substances are inherently carcinogenic, whereas others undergo bioactivation (such as metabolism by the P450 system) to produce reactive metabolites.

Certain complete carcinogens will produce malignant tumors through the multistep process without administration of a second chemical. Other carcinogens are only *initiators* and require subsequent action of a *promoter* in order to produce cancer. Most promoters are inactive unless there was prior exposure to an initiator; however, some promoters have induced cancer when used at high doses without an initiator.

There are many naturally occurring and synthetic carcinogens. Exposure to carcinogens can occur at work, in the diet, or from other environmental sources. Carcinogenesis can result from chronic exposure to low levels of certain carcinogens, and a long latent period may occur before clear manifestation of the disease. Cancer can also arise through exposure to ionizing radiation and certain cell-transforming viruses. Estimating potential carcinogenicity is a major concern in the registration of drugs, food additives, and pesticides, as well as in the control of toxic substances in research and manufacturing.

Genetic Carcinogens and Mutagenesis

Genetic carcinogens produce damage to DNA primarily through their interaction with the purine and pyrimidine bases found in the molecule. Mutations which affect only a single pair of bases in the DNA chain are known as gene or *point mutations*. Point mutations generally affect one single codon (the group of three bases which code for a single amino acid in protein synthesis) potentially causing substitution of one amino acid for another in the resulting protein. This change may or may not affect protein function, depending on its location in the molecule. Mutations which lead to the insertion or deletion of bases, however, disrupt the triplet code and can affect all downstream codons. Such an event is known as a *frame-shift mutation*, and is likely to block production of functional proteins by that gene (Figure 1).

It is the purine and pyrimidine bases which possess the critical nucleophilic sites where chemical changes such as *alkylation* (addition of an alkyl group) can occur. This reaction occurs when the nucleophilic atom of a nucleotide, such as guanine *N*-7 or *O*-6, attacks the electrophilic carbon of the alkylating agent (substrate) forming a covalent bond. If a nucleotide base (such as the purine base, gua-

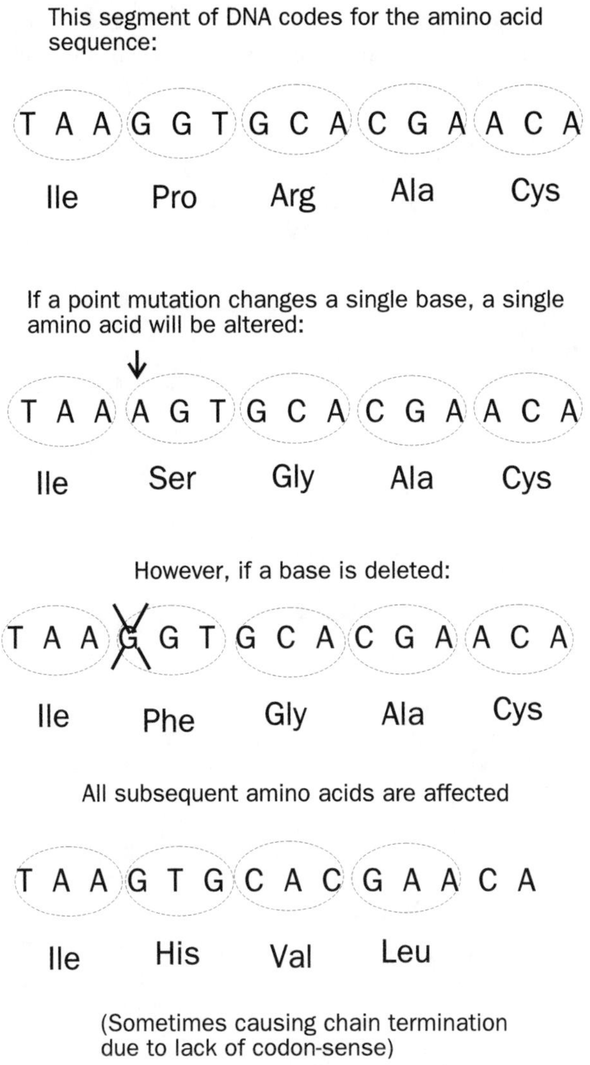

This segment of DNA codes for the amino acid sequence:

T A A G G T G C A C G A A C A

Ile   Pro   Arg   Ala   Cys

If a point mutation changes a single base, a single amino acid will be altered:

↓

T A A A G T G C A C G A A C A

Ile   Ser   Gly   Ala   Cys

However, if a base is deleted:

T A A G G T G C A C G A A C A

Ile   Phe   Gly   Ala   Cys

All subsequent amino acids are affected

T A A G T G C A C G A A C A

Ile   His   Val   Leu

(Sometimes causing chain termination due to lack of codon-sense)

Figure 1 A comparison between point mutations and frame shift mutations.

nine, for example) is alkylated, its ability to correctly pair with its complementary base (in this case cytosine) may be impaired. Thus, as DNA polymerase catalyses the synthesis of the complementary strand during DNA replication, an incorrect pyrimidine base (thymine, rather than cytosine) might be inserted, resulting in mutation (Figure 2).

Alkylating agents are one of the best defined categories of chemical carcinogen. One typical example of an alkylating agent is mustard gas, which was employed as a chemical weapon in World War I. This agent was first found to react with nucleotide bases of DNA *in vitro*. Then, as predicted, alkylated DNA was isolated from exposed mice. It was also found that the ability of various alkylating agents to induce cancer in mice was dose dependent, and was directly related to the degree of alkylation of mouse thymus DNA *in vivo*. Similar studies

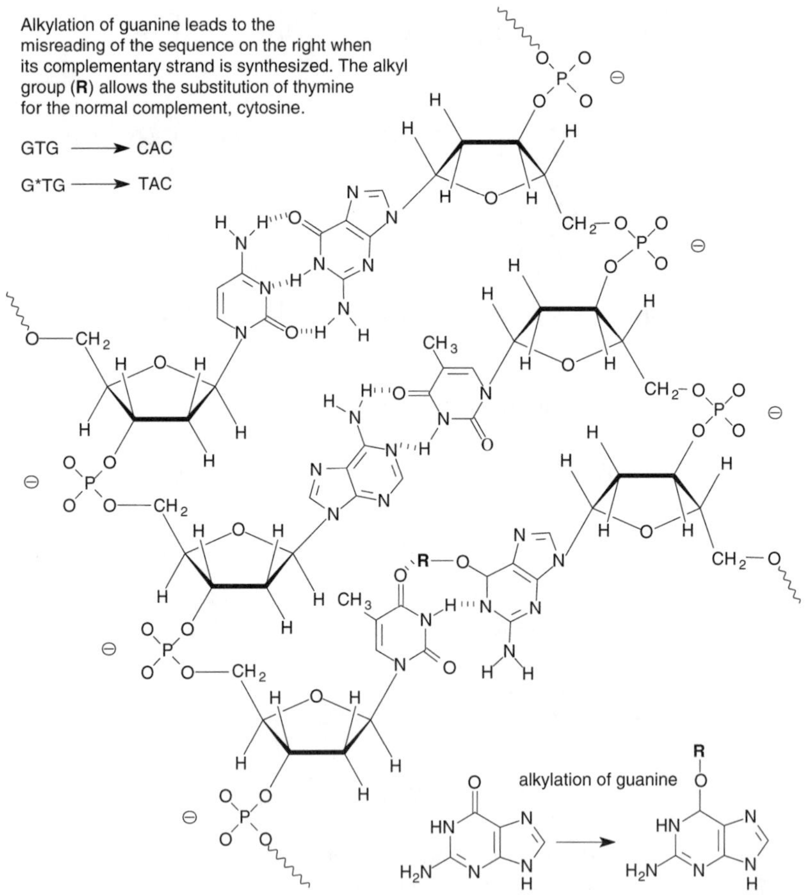

Figure 2   Alkylation of guanine.

have demonstrated that alkylation of DNA is better correlated with cancer development than alkylation of RNA or protein. This provides strong evidence that DNA is indeed the target for the reactions which can initiate carcinogenesis.

Another class of alkylating agents is the *polycyclic aromatic hydrocarbons (PAHs)*. Produced during the combustion of organic materials (for example, they are an important component of cigarette smoke), these compounds are metabolized by P450 through epoxidation to yield reactive metabolites. *N-nitroso compounds* are another example. These compounds are also found in cigarette smoke, and are potentially formed in the stomach when ingested nitrates combine with secondary amines.

PAHS
see also:
Reproductive toxicology
and teratology   *Ch. 6, p. 77*
PAHs   *Appendix, p. 244*

Other potentially chemically induced changes to DNA include *changes in chromosome structure*, e.g., breakage and rearrangement, or loss of genetic material. *Radiation* is a potent genetic carcinogen which can produce changes in chromosome structure. Other toxicants can potentially cause the *gain or loss of entire chromosomes*, although these toxicants usually do not act directly on the DNA, but instead act on other cellular components involved in cell division (e.g., spindle fibers).

Epigenetic Carcinogens

While genotoxic carcinogens such as alkylating agents are reactive with DNA, many other carcinogens are believed to produce cancer through epigenetic mechanisms, i.e., by affecting cellular regulation by mimicking hormones. One example of a compound which is likely to act in this way is *TCDD*. TCDD displays highly specific affinity to a cytosolic receptor protein. Upon binding of TCDD to this receptor, the complex moves to the nucleus, binds to a DNA receptor binding site, and induces the transcription of the gene for the enzyme arylhydro-

TCDD
see also:
Biotransformation   *Ch. 3, p. 20*
Immunotoxicology   *Ch. 12, p. 179*
Water pollution   *Ch. 15, p. 218*
TCDD   *Appendix, p. 245*

carbon hydroxylase (AH) along with several other genes. This may lead to promotion of cell division through actions on various regulating enzymes. TCDD may also act in synergy with carcinogens which require bioactivation, producing an increase in P450 levels and thus leading to increases in production of reactive metabolites. Finally, TCDD may promote development of cancer through its immunosuppressive effects.

Other potentially epigenetic carcinogens include promoters of cell division such as the *phorbol esters*, *hormones* such as estrogens, and *heavy metals*. The mechanism by which metals act as carcinogens is unclear. Some evidence indicates that they may in fact interact with DNA, but other evidence points toward inhibition of DNA repair mechanisms (more about repair later in this chapter).

MECHANISMS OF CARCINOGENESIS—ONCOGENES AND TUMOR SUPPRESSOR GENES

The Discovery of Oncogenes

The question of how changes to DNA can result in the neoplastic transformation of a cell is the key to understanding cancer. Initial clues to the answer came with the study of certain RNA tumor viruses, called acutely transforming retroviruses, which can cause cancer in animals. Using the enzyme reverse transcriptase (encoded in the RNA), the virus can produce DNA from its RNA. The DNA can then be inserted into the genome of the host. When the retroviral genes which were inserted into tumor cells were examined, some of them were found to resemble normal cellular genes of the host. These cancer-inducing genes were called *oncogenes* and the analogous (yet apparently inactive) genes in normal cells became known as *protooncogenes*. This discovery, which has led to many new molecular approaches to understanding carcinogenesis, earned the Nobel Prize for Bishop and Varmus.

Insertion of a viral oncogene, however, is not the only way in which cancer arises. It appears that cellular protooncogenes can be activated to become oncogenes themselves. Protooncogene activation to an oncogene can occur in several ways. For example, some cancer viruses lack oncogenes; however, they can exert a similar effect by disrupting a protooncogene through *insertional mutagenesis* (that is, by inserting the viral genome within the sequence of the protooncogene).

Yet in malignant tumor biopsy samples, activated oncogenes are found even without the involvement of RNA virus, indicating that other agents are capable of activating protooncogenes. Chemically induced mutations in the protooncogene or in areas of the genome which control its transcription may also initiate activation. Gene amplification, where multiple copies of a region of DNA are made, may also trigger activation and several known cases of activation are associated with chromosome aberration, such as the Philadelphia chromosome of leukemia. Altogether, oncogene activation has been associated with a number of various leukemias, carcinomas, and sarcomas.

Protooncogenes and Their Roles in Cell Function

Protooncogenes have been mapped throughout human genome and they are also found in many other organisms such as *Drosophila melanogaster*. Their evolutionary conservation suggests important roles in the normal life of the cell. Oncogenes are given three letter names, e.g., *src*, and those with both viral and eukaryotic homologues are denoted by prefix as either *v-src* for viral-*src* or *c-src* for cellular-*src*.

The process of cell growth and division, known as *mitogenesis*, is regulated by biochemical signals which are received, relayed through the cell, and regulate DNA transcription or replication. Protooncogenes encode various protein products associated with this signal transduction across the membrane, through the cytoplasm, and into the nucleus (Figure 3). These products affect mitogenesis and interactions between cells.

Among the chemical messengers which promote cell division are small- to medium-sized polypeptides called *growth factors* (one example is epidermal growth factor). Growth factors promote cell division by binding to selective receptors on the outer surface of the cell. Several oncogenes code for proteins which are related to growth factors. For example, platelet-derived growth factor (PDGF) β-chain is coded for by the oncogene *c-sis*, while similar fibroblast growth factor-like proteins are encoded by *int* and *hst* oncogenes.

Platelet-derived growth factor receptor (PDGF-R) is a *growth factor receptor* with tyrosine kinase activity, as are the products of the oncogenes *c-fms* and *c-kit*.

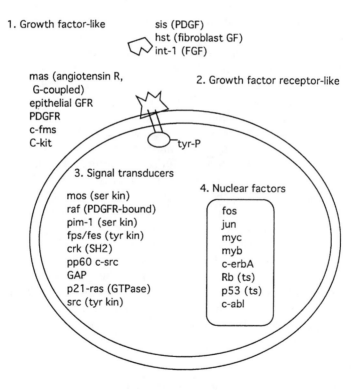

Figure 3   Cellular sites of protooncogene and tumor suppressor (ts) action.

These genes resemble tyrosine kinases from retroviral oncogenes, but they all produce proteins composed of three parts: a growth hormone receptor domain on the outer membrane surface, a single hydrophobic domain crossing the membrane, and an obligatory tyrosine kinase domain on the interior. Mutations which destroy the tyrosine kinase activity also block receptor signaling activity in these proteins. On the other hand, mutations in the transmembrane region can enhance cell transforming activity of the oncogenes suggesting a short circuiting of the signal through an unknown mechanism. Other oncogenes including *erb, ros,* and *met* are also associated with growth factor receptor tyrosine kinases. In addition, genes involved in differentiation of *Drosophila* such as *sevenless* and *torso,* have the characteristics of this class. In *sevenless* mutant fruit flies, one of eight photoreceptor cells of the ommatidium (compound eye) develops incorrectly to become a cone cell. The *sevenless* gene encodes a tyrosine kinase amino acid sequence similar to the oncogene *ros.*

Binding of growth factors to the growth factor receptor triggers autophosphorylation (self-phosphorylation) of tyrosines on the portion of the receptor inside the cell. The phosphorylation signal is then passed to cytosolic (nonreceptor) tyrosine kinases and other signal transducing proteins. The signal transducing proteins wrap tightly around the phosphorylated tyrosine, so that the phosphate groups on the tyrosine associate with SH_2 residues lying too deeply within the signal transducing molecule to be reached by other phosphorylated amino acid residues (such as serine or threonine).

Some cellular functions are mediated through a cascade of protein phosphorylation beginning with the growth factor receptor autophosphorylation just described. Oncogenes *src, abl, fgr, yes, fes, fps, sea, tck,* and *trk* all encode tyrosine kinases which catalyze protein phosphorylation on tyrosine residues. Serine/threonine kinases are produced by *raf, mos,* and *pim* oncogenes.

Analysis of the human carcinoma-associated *mas* oncogene has implicated another type of receptor—a neurotransmitter receptor—in mitogenesis. This oncogene encodes a receptor protein with seven hydrophobic, transmembrane domains and a lack of intrinsic tyrosine kinase activity. It is homologous to the receptor for the small peptide neurotransmitter, angiotensin. Signal transduction from these receptors depends on interaction with G proteins on the inner surface of the membrane. GTPases, such as *p21*, are products of *N-ras, H-ras,* and *K-ras.*

Other oncogene products are found in the cell nucleus. These include transcription factor AP-1, the product of *jun*, which interacts with the protein product of oncogene *fos* to form a protein heterodimer capable of regulating gene transcription. Oncogenes *myc, ski, ets, myb,* and *rel* also generate nuclear proteins. Nuclear oncogenes often contain a zinc-finger motif which is characteristic of proteins capable of interacting with DNA.

Tumor Suppressor Genes

Tumor suppressor genes are genes which limit cell proliferation and must be overcome in order for a developing tumor to progress. Like oncogenes, their mutated forms were also associated with tumors, so some were originally considered to be oncogenes. Like protooncogenes, tumor suppressors are critical cellular components as demonstrated by the lack of viable progeny from mice with *Rb-1* selectively deleted. Tumor suppressors can be considered guardians of the body against proliferation of deleterious cells. They can halt cell phase progression, activate postmitotic differentiation, or cause apoptosis (programmed cell death). For example, *p53* gene generates nuclear protein p53 which monitors for deleterious mutations and can shut down replication of cultured tumor cells when its concentration rises.

Development of a tumor generally requires that functional products of suppressor genes be negated by deletion or destructive mutation of both copies of the gene. It was recently observed, for example, that the tumor suppressor gene *APC* in colorectal tumors was usually mutated on both alleles. An indirect way to negate the action of these genes is by sequestrating the suppressor protein. For example, the oncogene *MDM2* produces MDM2, which binds to the tumor suppressor gene product p53. Gene amplification of *MDM2* in human sarcomas probably results in high concentrations of MDM2, which then removes p53 through binding. The negation of tumor suppressors, as contrasted with the positive activation of protooncogenes, is also supported by the observation that there are many different destructive mutation sites in p53 and in APC, but there are only a few mutations conferring activation of *ras*.

Examples of tumor suppressors are *p53* (found in many cancers), *DCC* (deleted in colon carcinoma), *APC* (adenomatous polyposis coli, also related to colorectal cancer), *Rb-1* (found in retinoblastoma), and *NF-1* (found in neurofibrosarcoma and Schwannoma—cancers of the nervous system).

EPIDEMIOLOGY OF CANCER

With approximately one-half million deaths annually, cancers are second only to heart diseases among causes of death in the U.S. Thus, cancers account for 20% of all fatalities in the U.S. Cancers are the leading cause of death in women in the U.S. Cancer incidence is higher among blacks than whites, and among males compared to females. Cancer incidence is much higher among the middle aged and elderly than among young people; this is most likely due to the multiple steps and latent period which characterize most forms of cancer.

Although genetic predisposition is recognized for certain populations in some forms of cancer, most cases appear to be due to environmental factors. For example, Japanese Americans living in Hawaii for several generations have a spectrum of cancer incidence which is very similar to other Hawaiian residents but unlike Japanese living in Japan. Other evidence includes sharp foci of lung cancer in the U.K. where high incidence was recorded near shipyards in which workers were exposed to asbestos. More than one half of cancer cases are related to diet and to use of tobacco; therefore, these diseases could be greatly reduced by changes in behavior and habits, such as lowering the intake of fatty foods.

More than half of the new cases of cancer in the U.S. and among most developed countries are found in lung, colon-rectum, breast, and prostate gland (Figure 4). Except for rectal cancer, incidence of these leading cancers has increased in the last two decades. Melanoma, occurring as 3% of new cancer cases, has nearly doubled. In Japan, which has a very low incidence of all cancers, stomach cancer is the most frequent form. This may be related to the relatively high intake of salt and nitrites in preserved foods in Japan.

Bronchogenic carcinomas (cancers of the lung), are increasing at a rapid rate, in both females and males, when compared to other cancers, and they exhibit a very high mortality. Recently, lung cancer surpassed breast cancer in mortality for women. Causal agents of bronchogenic carcinoma include occupational hazards such as asbestos in shipyard workers; however, the steep rise of incidence is likely a result of tobacco use.

Several forms of bronchogenic carcinoma occur and can be identified histologically and smokers exhibit greatly altered proportions among those forms (Figure 5). *Small cell carcinoma* is more common among smokers. Originating in areas of bronchial epithelium, small cell carcinoma tumors often produce hormones and biogenic amines, block the bronchial passages, and often invade other tissues. *Squamous cell carcinoma* often arises in the larger bronchi of the lung and is often preceded by damage and degeneration of the squamous epithelium (often following chronic exposure to pollution or smoking). Ciliated cells are lost and mucosal cells increase in number. It often invades adjacent tissues and nearby lymph nodes, and metastasis is likely. *Adenocarcinoma* is less common; however,

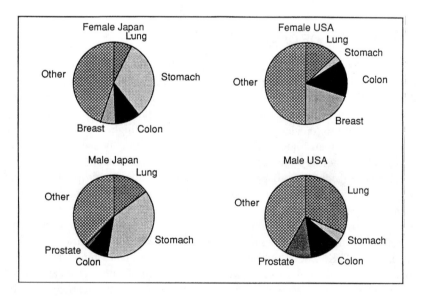

Figure 4   Incidence of various types of cancers in the U.S. and Japan.

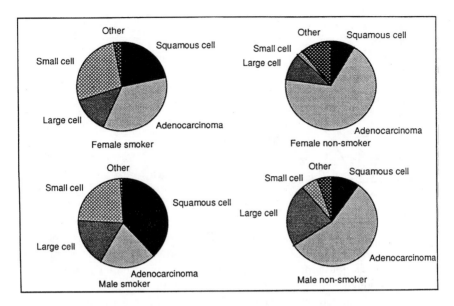

Figure 5   Types of lung cancer found in smokers and nonsmokers.

among nonsmokers it accounts for the majority of bronchogenic carcinoma cases. Adenocarcinomas usually originate peripherally in the bronchial tree, exhibiting a glandular form, but are less likely to involve the lymph nodes compared to squamous cell carcinomas. *Large cell carcinoma* also arises peripherally; it too commonly affects the lymph nodes. Small cell carcinoma occasionally occurs in a mixture with squamous cell carcinoma or with adenocarcinoma.

There has been much progress in the treatment or prevention of cancer of cervix, uterus, and stomach in recent years; however, lung and pancreatic cancer remain highly lethal.

PROTECTION AGAINST THE DEVELOPMENT OF CANCER

Fortunately, there are several intrinsic mechanisms which act to block the initiation, promotion, and progression of neoplasms. First, there are several enzymes which work to repair damage to DNA. *Methyltransferase* enzymes, for example, cleave methyl groups from guanine. *Excision repair systems* consist of *endonucleases* which open the DNA strand to allow removal of the damaged or mispaired base, *polymerases* which insert the correct base, and *ligases* which reseal the strand. Individuals with defects in these repair systems are much more susceptible to developing cancer than the general population. The immune system also provides surveillance. Abnormal surface proteins (called *tumor-specific antigens*) may appear on the surface of neoplastic cells, marking them for destruction

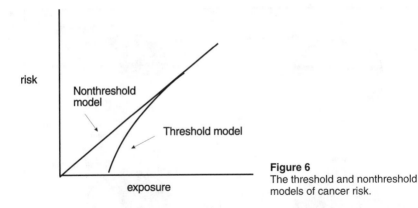

Figure 6
The threshold and nonthreshold
models of cancer risk.

by lymphocytes called *natural killer cells*. Cytotoxic T cells and a class of cells called *tumor-infiltrating lymphocytes* (TILs) also participate in tumor destruction. Evidence for the participation of the immune system in tumor destruction is strong. Individuals with disease-induced or deliberate (as in the case of organ transplantation) immunosuppression have a much higher risk of cancer than the general population. Also, physicians have recently had some success in treating cancer through immune system stimulation.

TESTING COMPOUNDS FOR CARCINOGENICITY

Based on the observation that many carcinogens are genetic in their mechanism of action, initial screening tests for carcinogenicity generally evaluate the mutagenicity of a compound. Screening tests should be simple and replicable, with few false negatives. One test which meets these criteria is an *in vitro* assay called the *Ames test*. In the Ames test, a mutant form of the bacteria *Salmonella typhinurium* is used. This mutant is unable to grow unless the nutrient histidine is supplied in the growth medium. Reversion to wild type (which does not require an external supply of histidine) can occur with base pair substitution or frame shift mutation at the appropriate location on the bacterial genome. Mutant bacteria are exposed to the potential mutagen/carcinogen, then cultured on a medium without histidine. Thus, the only colonies which will survive are those that arise from bacteria which have undergone mutation and reverted to wild type. Bacterial growth is compared between the test group and one or more control groups (which are unexposed to the potential mutagen/carcinogen). A positive control (a group which has been treated with a known mutagen) is often used. There are numerous variations on this test, some of which use mammalian cells. Another type of *in vitro* testing, *cytogenetic testing*, focuses on visual identification of chromosomal aberrations in populations of exposed cells.

One problem with the Ames test and similar *in vitro* tests is that compounds which require metabolic activation to produce mutagenic/carcinogenic metabolites may test negative. To remedy this, preparations of isolated mammalian liver smooth endoplasmic reticulum may be added to the test. This cytochrome P450-containing preparation (called the *S9* component) carries out metabolism of the test compound and thus allows testing of metabolites as well.

There are also a variety of *in vivo* test methods to determine carcinogenicity. Generally, testing is done using mice and rats, with routes of administration of the potential carcinogen chosen to most closely resemble the route by which human exposures would be expected to occur. In a typical chronic study, exposure to the potential carcinogen begins shortly after birth and continues for 1 to 2 years. At the end of the study, animals are examined and control and treated groups are compared with respect to survival, number of tumors, types of tumors, and onset time to development of tumors. Because incidence of background tumors may be high, high dosages and large group sizes may be necessary to demonstrate statistically significant differences between the treated and control groups.

The relationship between exposure to carcinogens and actual risk of developing cancer is controversial. Although there is evidence that the relationship may be linear at high exposure levels, it cannot be assumed that this is also true at low exposure levels, and the limits in sensitivity of testing methods make experimental verification difficult if not impossible. Some scientists believe that the exposure/risk curve is, in fact, linear; others, however, believe that there is a *threshold* exposure below which risk is negligible. Proponents of the threshold model argue that our food, water, and environment are replete with carcinogens and that without a threshold cancer rates would be much higher than they are. They also point to defense mechanisms such as detoxification reactions, DNA repair, and immune surveillance which should be able to cope with low-level exposures.

REFERENCES

Aaronson, S. A., Growth factors and cancer, *Science*, 254, 1146, 1991.

Balmain, A. and Brown, K., Oncogene activation in chemical carcinogenesis, *Adv. Cancer Res.*, 51, 147, 1988.

Bishop, J. M., The molecular genetics of cancer, *Nature*, 235, 305, 1987.

Bock, G. and Marsh, J., *Proto-oncogenes in Cell Development*, John Wiley & Sons, Chichester, 1990, 295.

Boguski, M. S., Bairoch, A., Attwood, T. K., and Michaels, George S., Proto-vav and gene expression, *Nature*, 358, 113, 1992.

Bourne, H. R. and Stryer, L., G proteins: the target sets the tempo, *Nature*, 358, 541, 1992.

Calabresi, P., Schein, P. S., and Rosenberg, S. A., *Medical Oncology*, Macmillan, New York, 1985, 1576.

Cohen, S. M. and Ellwein, L. B., Cell proliferation in carcinogenesis, *Science*, 249, 1007, 1990.

Downward, J., Signal transduction: Rac and Rho in tune, *Nature*, 359, 273, 1992.

Farmer, G., Bargonetti, J., Zhu, H., Friedman, P., Prywes, R., and Prives, C., Wild-type p53 activates transcription in vitro, *Nature*, 358, 83, 1992.

Harlow, E., Retinoblastoma: for our eyes only, *Nature*, 359, 270, 1992.

Harris, C. C. and Liotta, L. A., *Genetic Mechanisms in Carcinogenesis and Tumor Progression,* John Wiley & Sons, New York, 1990, 235.

Hausen, H. zur, Viruses in human cancers, *Science,* 254, 1167, 1991.

Henderson, B. E., Ronald, K., Ross, R. K., and Pike, M. C., Toward the primary prevention of cancer, *Science,* 254, 1131, 1991.

Hoffman, G. R., Genetic toxicology, in *Casarett and Doull's Toxicology: The Basic Science of Poisons,* Amdur, M. O., Doull, J., and Klaassen, C. D., Eds., Pergamon Press, New York, 1991, chap. 6.

Kaplan, D. R., Hempstead, B. L., Martin-Zanca, D., Chao, M. V., and Parada, L. F., The trk proto-oncogene product: a signal tranducing receptor for nerve growth factor, *Science,* 252, 554, 1991.

Lane, D. P., Cancer: p53, guardian of the genome, *Nature,* 358, 15, 1992.

Oliner, J. D., Kinzler, K. W., Meltzer, P. S., George, D. L., and Vogelstein, B., Amplification of a gene encoding a p53-associated protein in human sarcomas, *Nature,* 358, 80, 1992.

Papas, T. S., *Oncogenesis: Oncogenes in Signal Transduction and Cell Proliferation,* Portfolio Publishing Company, The Woodlands, TX, 1990, 343.

Pastan, I. and Fitzgerald, D., Recombinant toxins for cancer treatment, *Science,* 254, 1173, 1991.

Pavletich, N. P. and Pabo, C. O., Zinc finger-DNA recognition: crystal structure of a Zif268-DNA complex at 2.1 Å, *Science,* 252, 809, 1991.

Petsko, G. A., Signal transduction: fishing in Src-infested waters, *Nature,* 358, 625, 1992.

Powell, S. M., Zilz, N., Beazer-Barclay, Y., Bryan, T. M., Hamilton, S. R., Thibodeau, S. N., Vogelstein, B., and Kinzler, K. W., APC mutations occur early during colorectal tumorigenesis, *Nature,* 359, 235, 1992.

Roberts, L., More pieces in the dioxin puzzle, *Science,* 254, 377, 1991.

Roberts, L., Paint kit for cancer diagnosis, *Science,* 254, 378, 1991.

Robens, J. F., Piegorsch, W. W., and Schueler, R. L., Methods of testing for carcinogenicity, in *Principles and Methods of Toxicology,* Hayes, A. W., Ed., Raven Press, New York, 1989, chap. 9.

Simon, M. I., Strathmann, M. P., and Gautam, N., Diversity of G proteins in signal transduction, *Science,* 252, 802, 1991.

Sluyser, M., *Molecular Biology of Cancer Genes,* Ellis Horwood Limited, Chichester, 1990, 292.

Solomon, E., Colorectal cancer genes, *Nature,* 343, 412, 1990.

Solomon, E., Borrow, J., and Goddard, A. D. Chromosome aberrations and cancer, *Science,* 254, 1153, 1991.

Waksman, G., Kominos, D., Robertson, S. C., Pant, N., and Baltimore, D., Crystal structure of the phosphotyrosine recognition domain SH2 of V-src complexed with tyrosine-phosphorylated peptides, *Nature,* 358, 646, 1992.

Williams, C., *Cancer Biology and Management: An Introduction,* John Wiley & Sons, Chichester, 1990.

Williams, G. M. and Weisburger, J. H., Chemical carcinogenesis, in *Casarett and Doull's Toxicology: The Basic Science of Poisons,* Amdur, M. O., Doull, J., and Klaassen, C. D., Eds., Pergamon Press, New York, 1991.

6

REPRODUCTIVE TOXICOLOGY AND TERATOLOGY

The functions of reproduction and development are complex, and involve many relatively unique cellular level processes. As such, the effects of toxicants on the process of reproduction and on developing organisms may be quite different from the effects of the same toxicant on other systems in the adult organism. This chapter first reviews a few basics, then considers the effects of toxicants on reproductive function (the production of eggs in the female and sperm in the male) and then proceeds on to effects of toxicants on developing organisms.

BASIC PROCESSES IN REPRODUCTION AND DEVELOPMENT— CELL DIVISION

Cell division plays a major role in both reproduction and development. The two basic types of cell division are (1) *mitosis*, where a single cell divides to form two identical daughter cells, and (2) *meiosis*, where daughter cells are produced which have only one instead of two copies of each chromosome.

During their lifetime, somatic cells (cells not involved in the formation of eggs or sperm) move through various stages in what is known as the *cell cycle* (Figure 1). Many cells spend virtually their entire lifetime in *interphase*. During the G_0 phase of interphase, cells carry out their normal functions. Cells which are preparing to divide move from the G_0 phase to the G_1 phase, where duplication of organelles and other cytoplasmic constituents occurs. Cells may spend from only a few hours to several months in this phase. During the next phase, the S phase (which lasts several hours), the cell makes a copy of its DNA. DNA in eukaryotic cells is, of course, found in the form of *chromatin*, long strands of DNA wrapped around proteins called histones. During DNA replication, the hydrogen bonds which bind together the two complementary strands of the DNA in each chromosome are disrupted, and the two strands separate. Enzymes called *DNA polymerases* and *ligases* then link together free DNA nucleotides to form a *new* complementary strand for each of the original strands (Figure 2). The result is that the cell now contains two copies of each stretch of chromatin.

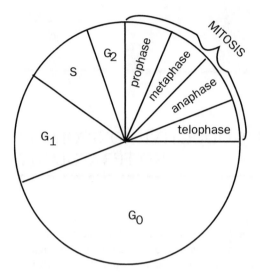

Figure 1
The cell cycle.

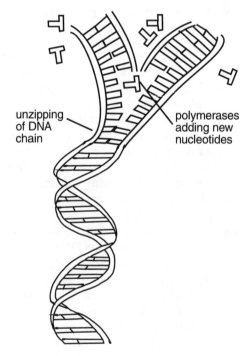

Figure 2
Semiconservative replication of DNA.

After a short period of protein synthesis (the G_2 phase), the cell enters the first stage of mitosis, which is *prophase* (Figure 3). At the beginning of prophase, the DNA coils up tightly to form the visible structures known as *chromosomes*. A chromosome consists of the two identical copies of the DNA made during the S phase (each of which is called a *chromatid*) held together at a point called the *centromere*. The two pairs of microtubular structures called *centrioles* move to opposite ends of the cell and *spindle fibers* form between the two pairs.

With the disappearance of the nuclear envelope, the cell moves into the second stage, which is *metaphase*. During metaphase, the chromosomes move to the center of the cell and attach to the spindle fibers. In the third stage, *anaphase*, each pair of chromatids separate and are pulled by the spindle fibers toward opposite ends of the cell. In the final stage, *telophase*, the nucleus reappears, the chromosomes uncoil, and the process of *cytokinesis*, the division of the cytoplasm, is completed. The end result is two daughter cells with the identical genetic makeup of the parent cell.

Cells which are to form eggs or sperm must go through a different process. Human cells contain 23 pairs of chromosomes: 22 autosomal pairs, and 1 pair of chromosomes which determine the sex of the individual. The two chromosomes

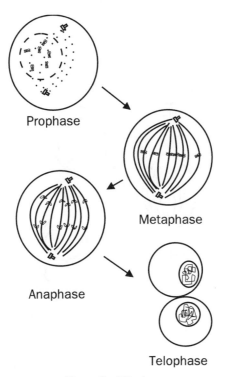

Prophase

Metaphase

Anaphase

Telophase

Figure 3 Mitosis.

which makeup one of these *homologous* pairs of autosomal chromosomes contain the same basic genes, and yet are not identical. Any given gene may exist in two or more variations called *alleles*. Thus, each of an individual's cells has two copies of each gene, and these copies may be either identical or different alleles. The assortment of alleles possessed by an individual is known as that individual's *genotype*. In the case of the sex chromosomes, there are two distinctive forms: the *X chromosome* and the *Y chromosome*. Individuals with two X chromosomes have a female genotype, while individuals with one X and one Y chromosome have a male genotype.

Cells with the normal number of pairs of chromosomes are described as *diploid*. In order for fusion of egg and sperm to produce a normal diploid zygote, each must contribute half the normal complement of chromosomes. Egg and sperm cells are, in fact, *haploid* (i.e., containing only one of each chromosome). Thus, in a zygote, one chromosome of each pair is contributed by the egg, and the other is contributed by the sperm.

Meiosis is the process by which haploid egg and sperm cells are created from diploid stem cells (Figure 4). Meiosis consists of a series of two divisions: meiosis I and meiosis II. Following duplication of cellular constituents (includ-

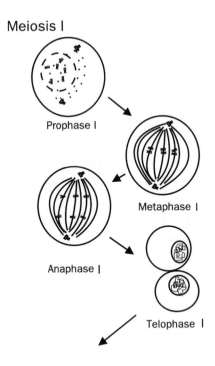

Figure 4   Meiosis.

ing DNA), such as precedes mitosis, the cell enters meiosis I. The stages of meiosis I are similar to the stages of mitosis *except* that when the chromosomes line up along the midline of the cell, they line up in homologous pairs. During this time, homologous chromosomes may also exchange genetic material (a process called *crossing over*) which can result in new combinations of alleles on a chromosome. Then, during anaphase I the homologous chromosomes separate and move to opposite ends of the cell. Thus each of the two resulting daughter cells is haploid. In meiosis II, each of these cells divides through a process virtually identical to mitosis to produce two identical haploid daughters each (a total of four haploid cells).

THE MALE REPRODUCTIVE SYSTEM

The formation of sperm occurs within organs called the *testes*, in tubules called *seminiferous tubules* (Figure 5). The process begins at puberty, and is regulated by the steroid hormone *testosterone* which is produced by interstitial cells that lie between the tubules. Secretion of testosterone is itself regulated by the pituitary hormone *luteinizing hormone* (LH). Another pituitary hormone, *follicle stimulating hormone* (FSH), is also important in spermatogenesis. Release of these pituitary hormones is, in turn, regulated by *gonadotropin releasing factor* (GnRF), which is released by the hypothalamus. The presence of testosterone produces a negative feedback effect, inhibiting the release of GnRF by the hypothalamus. When testosterone levels decline, though, GnRF release occurs.

The process of spermatogenesis begins when diploid cells called spermatogonia divide by mitosis, forming daughter cells. Some of these cells will remain as spermatogonia and some will mature into *primary spermatocytes*. Each primary spermatocyte undergoes meiosis I to form two haploid *secondary spermatocytes*, which each complete meiosis II, dividing to form two *spermatids* each.

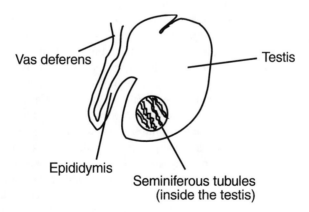

Figure 5 The testes.

Cytokinesis during these divisions is not completed, however, so the spermatids remain connected through their cytoplasm. Under the influence of the Sertoli cells, the spermatids separate, and mature into *spermatozoons*, which then migrate to the vas deferens where they continue to mature and eventually are stored for release. The whole process takes about 80 days.

Sperm stored in the vas deferens can remain active for several weeks. During the process of ejaculation, these sperm are ejected through the urethra, along with fluid from glands such as the seminal vesicles, bulbourethrals, and the prostate. Typically, a few milliliters of this *semen* is released, containing upwards of 100 million spermatozoa. Normal reproductive function is often assessed by examining the concentration of sperm in semen, as well as the motility and histologic appearance of individual spermatozoons.

THE EFFECTS OF TOXICANTS
ON THE MALE REPRODUCTIVE SYSTEM

The testes are afforded some degree of protection against toxicants by what is termed the *blood-testis barrier*. Tight junctions between the Sertoli cells in the seminiferous tubules form a barrier which prevents many substances from entering the areas where spermatozoons are developing. The testes also have metabolic capability in the form of cytochrome P450 activity, and the cells which will give rise to spermatozoa have at least some DNA repair capabilities.

There are several sites involved in the process of spermatogenesis at which toxicants may act. Because the process is under hormonal control, interference with the secretion of GnRF, LH, FSH, or testosterone could have an impact. *Estrogens* and *progestins* block spermatogenesis by suppressing LH and FSH, and thus testosterone secretion. *Anabolic steroids* are synthetic drugs which were developed in an attempt to separate the anabolic (muscle building) effects of steroids from the androgenic (reproductive) effects. This separation is, in fact, unachievable, since both reproductive and muscle tissues seem to contain the identical type of androgen receptor. These synthetic steroids may, however, lower testosterone levels (probably through feedback inhibition of GnRF, LH, and FSH) and suppress spermatogenesis. Other undesirable side effects of anabolic steroids include hepatotoxicity, behavioral changes, and potential shortening of stature in prepubertal males through premature termination of long bone growth.

These hormonal compounds, along with others that either block binding of testosterone to the androgen receptor or inhibit enzymes involved in testosterone synthesis, have been suggested as potential *male birth control agents*. Unfortunately, it is difficult to *completely* block spermatogenesis reliably. In addition, many of these drugs also produce unacceptable side effects such as irreversibility of effects, depression of libido, or toxicity to other organ systems.

Toxicants which interfere with cell division, such as alkylating agents (which damage DNA) and antimetabolites (which inhibit nucleotide biosynthesis), can directly inhibit sperm production. Likewise, physical agents such as *x-rays* and other forms of ionizing radiation probably cause decreases in spermatogenesis through effects on dividing cells.

Another toxicant, the pesticide *dibromochloropropane* (DBCP), caused destruction of seminiferous tubule epithelium in exposed workers, inhibiting spermatogenesis either through what may have been either effects on primary spermatogonia or through effects on Sertoli cells. The mechanism of action of DBCP in either case may be through inhibition of oxidative phosphorylation. Other toxicants which may affect energy metabolism include *dinitrobenzene, dinitrotoluene* (DNT), and various *phthalates* (plasticizing compounds).

Heavy metals such as *lead* and *cadmium* are well-known reproductive toxicants. Exposure to lead has been associated with infertility as well as with chromosomal damage in sperm. Cadmium can cause testicular necrosis, probably by decreasing blood flow to the testes. *Ethanol* causes delays in testicular development and may affect supporting cells. Other male reproductive toxins include the pesticides *kepone* and *DDT*, the solvent *carbon disulfide*, and even *tobacco* (smokers have higher percentages of abnormal sperm than nonsmokers).

CADMIUM
see also:

Cardiovascular toxicology	*Ch. 8, p. 111*
Renal toxicology	*Ch.11, p. 165*
Water pollution	*Ch. 15, p. 232*
Cadmium	*Appendix, p. 235*

LEAD
see also:

Cardiovascular toxicology	*Ch. 8, p. 114*
Neurotoxicology	*Ch. 9, p. 140, 143*
Immunotoxicology	*Ch. 12, p. 180*
Water pollution	*Ch. 15, p. 222*
Lead	*Appendix, p. 239*

THE FEMALE REPRODUCTIVE SYSTEM

The same basic hormonal system which controls reproduction in the male also controls reproduction in the female. GnRF is released by the hypothalamus, initiating secretion of LH and FSH by the pituitary. In the female, though, the effects of LH and FSH are to promote the syntheses of the *estrogens* and *progestins*. These hormones participate in a complex feedback system which regulates the release of GnRF, LH, and FSH.

The pair of organs in which egg production takes place are the *ovaries* (Figure 6). Early in development, several million oogonia develop in each

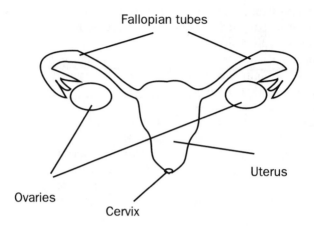

Figure 6   The ovaries, fallopian tubes, and uterus.

ovary. These oogonia barely begin the process of meiosis and then stop in prophase I. At this stage they are called *primary oocytes*. They are still diploid, and they remain in an arrested state until many years later, when puberty begins. The primary oocytes along with the cells which surround them are called *primary follicles*.

Many primary oocytes degenerate, so that at puberty each ovary probably contains a few hundred thousand primary follicles. Then, release of the hormone FSH each month (as part of the menstrual cycle) stimulates some follicles to grow into larger *secondary follicles*. One secondary follicle each month will continue to grow, while the primary oocyte within completes the first part of meiosis to become a haploid *secondary oocyte*. (The secondary oocyte receives most of the cytoplasm; the other, much smaller daughter cell is called a *polar body* and ultimately disintegrates.) The secondary oocyte continues to grow along with the follicle, which fills with fluid secreted by the follicular cells. The structure is now known as a *tertiary follicle*. A surge in the hormone LH at about the fourteenth day of the menstrual cycle stimulates release of the secondary oocyte and some of its surrounding follicular cells. It enters the fallopian tubes (where fertilization, if it is to occur, takes place) and begins the trip to the uterus. The empty follicle becomes the *corpus luteum*, secreting estrogen and progesterone until it eventually decays. If pregnancy occurs, a hormone secreted by the developing embryo (human chorionic gonadotropin) maintains the corpus luteum until the placenta develops and takes over the secretion of these hormones.

The uterus is a pear-shaped organ where development of the fertilized egg occurs. Under the influence of estrogens and progestins the lining of the uterus (the *endometrium*) undergoes a monthly cycle of changes, first proliferating to produce a thick zone where the developing zygote can implant, then if fertilization does not occur, shedding this newly developed tissue during *menstruation*.

THE EFFECTS OF TOXICANTS
ON THE FEMALE REPRODUCTIVE SYSTEM

As in the male, toxicants which interfere with the hormonal control of reproduction can impair fertility. Anesthetics, analgesics, and other drugs which interfere with either neuronal or hormonal control of hypothalamic or pituitary function prevent ovulation. *Birth control drugs* such as oral contraceptives, as well as injectable (Depo-Provera) and implantable (Norplant) contraceptives also act on this hormonal system. These drugs contain a mixture of estrogen and progestins which inhibit the release of FSH and LH and thus inhibit ovulation. Side effects associated with these drugs include some increase in risk of thromboembolism (obstruction of a blood vessel by a blood clot), myocardial infarction, and stroke. These risks increase with age and with the presence of contributing factors such as smoking and underlying cardiovascular disease. There is some evidence that users of these drugs may also experience slightly increased risk for breast, vaginal, and uterine cancers; risk for ovarian cancer, however, may actually decline.

Cytotoxic substances such as *antineoplastic agents, heavy metals, polycyclic aromatic hydrocarbons*, or *radiation* may damage oocytes, particularly in adult women. The effects of such agents depend on which stage of oocyte development is affected. Effects on mature secondary oocytes will lead to temporary infertility, with fertility being restored as new secondary oocytes develop. Partial destruction of primary oocytes, however, may lead not to immediate infertility, but to early onset of menopause (which occurs when the total pool of primary oocytes in the ovary falls below a minimum number). Total destruction of primary oocytes, though, will lead to infertility as well as to premature menopause. Nonlethal effects of these agents on oocytes include DNA damage which may lead to genetic defects in offspring.

Some of these cytotoxic toxicants (polycyclic aromatic hydrocarbons, for example) must be metabolized in order to produce toxicity. This activation can occur in the ovary, as cytochrome P450 and other enzymes involved in xenobiotic metabolism are found in ovarian tissues. Toxic PAH metabolites

---

POLYCYCLIC AROMATIC HYDROCARBONS
see also:
   Carcinogenesis   *Ch. 5, p. 59*
   PAHs   *Appendix, p. 244*

---

destroy primary oocytes, which is one possible explanation for the observation that exposure to cigarette smoke (which contains PAHs) may lead to premature menopause.

Many other toxicants, including some *pesticides, chlorinated hydrocarbon solvents*, and *aromatic solvents* have also been reported to interfere with female reproductive capacity.

THE PROCESS OF DEVELOPMENT

Fertilization generally occurs in the fallopian tubes when a spermatozoon penetrates the outer covering of the oocyte and activates it. At that time, the second stage in meiosis is completed, forming the oocyte and also forming a second polar body. Following penetration, the nuclei of the spermatozoon and the oocyte fuse, forming a *zygote*.

The single-celled zygote then enters into a period of rapid cell division, or *cleavage* and eventually forms a hollow ball of cells called a *blastocyst* (Figure 7). By this time (a few days after fertilization), the blastocyst has passed from the fallopian tubes into the uterus where it implants in the uterine lining. The outer cells of the blastocyst (called the *trophoblast*) divide, grow, penetrate, and breakdown the endometrial tissues, releasing nutrients which can be used by the inner cell mass from which the embryo will develop.

Meanwhile, the inner cell mass separates from the trophoblast, and a fluid-filled cavity (the *amniotic cavity*) forms between them. The cells of the inner cell mass form an oval sheet called the *blastodisc*. By the end of the second week the differentiation of cells (probably triggered by differences in cytoplasmic constituents and cellular environments) leads to the formation of three distinct layers: the *ectoderm*, which will form the epidermis as well as the epithelial linings of oral, nasal, anal and vaginal cavities, nervous tissue, and some endocrine organs; the *mesoderm*, which will form muscle and connective tissues, vascular endothelium and lymph vessels, the lining of some body cavities, the reproductive and urinary systems, and some other endocrine organs; and the *endoderm*, which becomes the epithelial lining of the gastrointestinal, respiratory, and urinary tracts.

Other tissues become the *extraembryonic membranes*, serving to protect, nourish, and support the developing embryo (Figure 8). One of these is the *yolk*

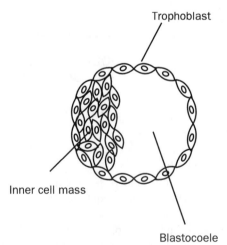

Trophoblast

Inner cell mass

Blastocoele

Figure 7   The blastocyst.

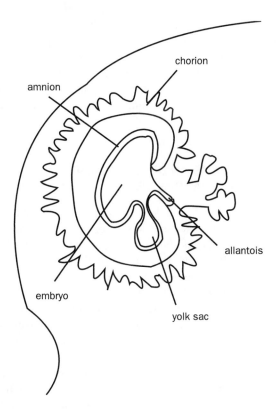

Figure 8 The extraembryonic membranes.

sac, which provides nourishment in some other species and serves in humans as the source for germ cells (cells which will become egg and sperm) and cells which will form the primitive gut. The *amnion* is an ectodermal and mesodermal membrane that encloses the developing embryo and amniotic fluid, and the *allantois* is involved in formation of fetal blood vessels, blood cells, and the bladder. The *chorion*, together with the trophoblast forms the *placenta*. Blood flows into the placenta through the umbilical arteries, and close juxtaposition of branches of these vessels with maternal blood circulating through cavities in the placenta allows the interchange of oxygen, nutrients, and waste materials through the process of diffusion. The placenta also produces estrogen, progesterone, and other hormones which help maintain the uterine lining, and thus the pregnancy.

By the fourth week, the longitudinal axis of the embryo develops in the form of the *primitive streak*, a thickened band along the midline of the blastodisc. During the next few weeks the rudiments of the nervous system develop, arm and leg buds develop, and the basic structures of most organ systems are formed. At this time, the production of testosterone by the embryonic testes initiates the steps which will result in the development of a male phenotype. (In the absence of testosterone, a female phenotype will develop regardless of genotypic sex.) By the end of 8 weeks the embryo is quite well developed, and is referred to as a *fetus*. Development and growth continues throughout the fetal period, and for some systems (such as the nervous system, for example) development even continues postnatally.

EFFECTS OF TOXICANTS ON DEVELOPMENT: TERATOGENS AND TERATOGENESIS

Teratology is the study of birth defects—structural or functional abnormalities that are present at birth. In humans, it is estimated that the presence of abnormalities leads to the spontaneous abortion of somewhere between 25 and 50% of all pregnancies, and birth defects occur in up to 10 to 15% of all live births. Of course, many of these problems may be caused by random genetic errors, but some are caused by environmental factors.

A *teratogen* is an environmental agent which produces birth defects. Common types of effects of teratogens on developing organisms include structural malformations, growth retardation, and death. Whether or not exposure to a teratogen produces a birth defect depends on several different factors. Two of the most important factors are dose or exposure level, and timing of exposure. There are other factors involved as well, many of which we do not yet understand. For example, prenatal exposure of a litter of rat pups to a teratogen may produce severe defects in some pups, milder defects in others, and no effects at all in a few. Reasons for this may include "microdifferences" in intrauterine conditions (causing, for example, some pups to be exposed to higher levels of the teratogen than others), variations in the state of development of different pups in the litter, or even genetic variations in susceptibility between pups.

Effects of Dose or Exposure Level on Teratogenicity

First, as with any toxicant, the actual dose or exposure level is an important factor. During pregnancy, such physiological changes as increased absorption of substances through the gastrointestinal tract, increases in lung tidal volume, and increases in blood flow to the skin all may enhance absorption of environmental toxicants. Also, as maternal blood volume increases, concentrations of the plasma protein albumin decrease, leading to fewer binding sites for toxicants, and a greater tendency for those toxicants to enter tissues. Counteracting this, however, is an increase in rate of renal excretion.

The placenta itself fails to provide much of a barrier to transfer of toxicants between the maternal and fetal compartments. Substances which are lipid soluble, small, and neutral in charge diffuse easily through the placenta. Other substances may cross by means of facilitated diffusion or active transport mechanisms. Metals (cadmium, for example) may also accumulate in the placenta.

Xenobiotic metabolism of toxicants is thought to occur mostly in maternal tissues or the placenta, as the levels of many enzymes which participate in both Phase I and Phase II bio-transformation are quite low in

XENOBIOTIC METABOLISM
see also:
   Biotransformation   *Ch. 3, p. 21*

developing organisms (in humans, P450 levels at midgestation are less than half the adult levels). Prenatal levels of P450 do, however, increase on exposure to inducers such as phenobarbital. Placental biotransformation activities although low, also are inducible (exposure to polycyclic aromatic hydrocarbons, as contained in cigarette smoke, significantly increases P450-A1 activity).

In general, as exposure levels increase, so does the severity of the teratogenic effect. Some teratogens produce only structural defects at low levels of exposure, but may be lethal at higher levels. Others may produce a range of effects from structural defects to lethality at the same exposure level. Maternal toxicity may or may not occur at exposure levels sufficient to produce birth defects. Thus, in many cases, exposures which would not threaten the health of the mother may be quite hazardous to the developing child.

Effects of Timing of Exposure on Teratogenicity

Because a variety of events occur at so many different times during the prenatal period, it stands to reason that the timing of exposure to a teratogen is critical in determining the potential effects. Exposure during the early stages (prior to implantation) is most likely to lead to embryonic death. Exposure during the late stages (in humans, the third trimester) is most likely to lead to growth retardation. It is during the middle stage, organogenesis, that exposure is most likely to lead to structural defects. Exposure to a teratogen during the *critical period* for a particular organ system may lead to malformations in that system. For example, exposure to the rubella virus during the first 8 weeks of pregnancy frequently produces defects of the visual and cardiovascular systems, while exposure during weeks 8 to 12 leads to hearing impairment. Critical periods in humans may vary in length from as long as several weeks to as short as a day.

Examples of Teratogens

One case which illustrates the importance of critical periods is the case of the drug *Thalidomide*. Used to treat nausea during early pregnancy ("morning sickness"),

THALIDOMIDE
see also:
   Thalidomide   *Appendix, p. 246*

this lipophilic drug easily crossed the placenta to cause the rare birth defects pho-comelia (severe shortening of the limbs) and amelia (lack of limbs) in several thousand children. Other effects included malformations of the cardiovascular, renal, and other systems. Because the drug was not approved for use in the U.S., most cases occurred in Europe and Japan. The drug was taken during the first 3 months of gestation (the time when morning sickness is typically the most severe), a time period which includes the critical period for limb development (weeks 7 to 8). Part of the reason why this drug was allowed on the market, was that mice and rats (the species in which most developmental tests were carried out) are relatively resistant to thalidomide teratogenicity.

A controversial prescription drug currently on the market is the drug *isotretinoin* (trade name Accutane). Although effective in the treatment of severe cystic acne in adults, it is also a potent teratogen, causing craniofacial, thymus, cardiac, and neurological defects. In spite of label warnings, educational programs, and pregnancy testing, some affected children are born each year. While many people would prefer to see this drug taken off the market, its effectiveness in dermatologic treatment makes such a decision difficult. This is an excellent example of a regulatory risk–benefit decision.

DES
see also:
   DES   ***Appendix, p. 237***

Another historic example was the use of the drug diethylstilbestrol (DES) to prevent potential miscarriage (a use for which it has been shown to be ineffective). Interference of this drug with normal reproductive tract development (particularly during weeks 6 to 16) led to structural and functional abnormalities of the reproductive tract in both DES-exposed daughters and sons. The problems associated with DES use were first noted when an unusually large number of cases of vaginal cancer (a cancer most often seen in older women) were seen in young women at Massachusetts General Hospital. There are other agents (other chemicals as well as radiation) which may also increase the risk of cancer in prenatally exposed offspring.

ETHANOL
see also:
   Neurotoxicology   ***Ch. 9, p. 143***
   Hepatotoxicology   ***Ch. 10, p. 155***
   Ethanol   ***Appendix, p. 237***

For some systems, such as the nervous system, critical periods extend throughout development. One teratogen with significant effects on this system is *ethanol. Fetal alcohol syndrome (FAS)* is a group of related effects including craniofacial abnormalities, growth retardation, and mental retardation which result from intrauterine exposure to ethanol. Severity of abnormalities seems to increase with increases in exposure levels. It is not certain whether there is a "safe" level of alcohol consumption during pregnancy, but risk of craniofacial and neurological abnormalities rises with the consumption of 2 oz. of ethanol per day, and risk of growth retardation rises with consumption of 1 oz/day. *Cocaine* use, also, has been associated with various abnormalities, including neurological problems and developmental deficits which may persist throughout life.

A number of heavy metals are also teratogens. *Cadmium*, as mentioned before, accumulates in the placenta and can cause fetal death through placental damage. Prenatal *lead* exposure may lead to neurological dysfunction, as does *methylmercury*.

METHYLMERCURY see also:	
Neurotoxicology	*Ch. 9, p. 142*
Renal toxicology	*Ch. 11, p. 165*
Water pollution	*Ch. 15, p. 222*
Mercury	*Appendix, p. 239*

Mechanisms of Teratogenicity

Not much is known about the biochemical mechanism of action of many teratogens, perhaps because there are so many gaps in our knowledge of the biochemical and cellular aspects of development. Of course, any agent that interferes with cell division is likely to damage developing organisms, where rates of cell division are very high. High levels of these compounds during organogenesis may produce organ malformations; lower levels may result in development of structurally normal, but smaller organs.

Probably more is known about the mechanisms involved in the production of *cleft palate* than for any other structural abnormality. The palate is formed by growth and fusion of maxillary and palatine process, an event involving cell division, migration, programmed cell death, and other complex processes. Cleft palate occurs when this process is disrupted. One toxicant known to be capable of producing cleft palate is *TCDD*, and it appears to do so by binding to proteins in the cytosol and blocking the programmed cell death necessary for normal palatal development. Exposure to high levels of *glucocorticoids* also causes cleft palate. Interaction of glucocorticoids with the glucocorticoid receptors in the maxillary cells inhibits cell growth.

Neurological effects of teratogens may be produced by many different mechanisms. Because the increased permeability of the fetal blood-brain barrier allows greater access to toxicants, the fetal brain may be susceptible to a wider range of insults than the adult brain. And, there are many specialized steps in neurological development which can potentially be disrupted by toxicants, including the development of neurotransmitters and receptors. Evidence indicates that these systems must be functioning properly in order for innervation to proceed correctly.

Thalidomide has been hypothesized to directly damage developing limb tissue or to interfere with communication between that tissue and surrounding tissues. DES seems to lead to failure of tissues from a temporary structure called the

Mullerian duct to either transform into normal tissues (in women) or to degenerate (in men). Cocaine potentiates the effects of norepinephrine (a neurotransmitter found in the sympathetic branch of the autonomic nervous system) by blocking reuptake. Because norepinephrine stimulates blood vessels to contract, this may lead to decreases in blood flow to the fetus, causing hypoxia. Norepinephrine also stimulates contraction of uterine smooth muscle, perhaps causing the tendency for premature labor observed in cocaine-use cases.

TESTING FOR REPRODUCTIVE AND DEVELOPMENTAL TOXICITY

Human Assessment

Reproductive and developmental toxicity assessment involves both the identification of problems in humans, and also investigations involving laboratory animals. In humans, reproductive history, sperm count (the concentration of sperm in the semen) and normality of sperm, and hormone levels in the blood are typically used to assess male reproductive functioning. In females, also, reproductive history is an important tool for assessing human fertility. In addition, x-rays of the uterus and fallopian tubes can identify structural abnormalities, and measurement of serum hormone levels, changes in body temperature, and other indicators can be used to evaluate for the presence or absence of ovulation.

Testing of Laboratory Animals—General Principles

A number of factors must be considered in developing tests for reproductive toxicity and teratogenicity involving laboratory animals. Because of interspecies differences in developmental pathways, xenobiotic metabolism, etc., the choice of species to be used in the test is critical. Hamsters, mice, and rats are common choices, due in part to their short gestation times (a purely practical advantage), but rabbits are also used, as are primates.

The route of administration for a toxicant should be similar to any routes for human exposure, and may include injection, intubation, inhalation, or delivery in food or water. Due to variations in food and water consumption, however, it is difficult to deliver a precise dose through this last route. Normally, multiple dose levels and a control (as well as solvent control, if necessary) are used, with dosages ranging from near the no-effect level to near the lethal level. In the case of teratology studies, exposure should continue throughout the length of the gestational period, especially during organogenesis.

In assessing male reproductive toxicity in laboratory animals, testicular weights are frequently used. Histological analyses of testicular cells and other cells of the male reproductive tract may also be useful in pinpointing targets of toxicants. Semen analysis can include sperm counts, studies of sperm motility, and sperm morphology (abnormalities in head shape, tail length, etc.). The ability of sperm to penetrate and fertilize an egg *in vitro* can also be studied.

Fertility profiles can be developed through regular mating of a toxicant-exposed male with a number of females followed by calculation of the percentage of females impregnated. During these matings, reproductive behavior can also be observed. Offspring from these matings are then studied for evidence of genetic defects.

In female laboratory animals, similar tests are used. Fertility profiles would involve mating of treated females, observation of mating behavior, assessment of the outcome of mating, and possibly evaluation of offspring. Likewise, histological evaluation of reproductive and endocrine organs is also used.

In Vitro Testing

Very young rat or mouse embryos (from conception up to the point where placental formation occurs) can be maintained in culture, exposed to teratogens, and observed for changes in normal development. Organs removed during organogenesis can also be cultured, as can cells or groups of cells. Some nonmammalian cell culture systems are also used in research and testing. These include cells derived from *Drosophila* (fruit fly) eggs, hydra cells, and *Xenopus* (an amphibian) embryos.

Established Procedures for Testing

Both the FDA and EPA have established procedures for evaluating reproductive and developmental toxicity. Standard FDA test protocols include:

Segment I: Assesses reproductive functions in male and female
Segment II: Assesses developmental toxicity
Segment III: Assesses peri- and postnatal toxicity

Other standard protocols include the *single generation reproduction test*, when both males or females or both are treated before and during mating. Gestation is allowed to proceed; the female nurses the litter for 3 weeks then all animals are killed and examined for abnormalities. The *multigeneration reproduction test* involves exposure of a parental generation (male and female) through gestation, continued exposure of their offspring (the F1 generation) through mating and gestation, and then exposure of the next generation (the F2) through weaning.

REFERENCES

Collins, T. F. X., Current protocols in teratology and reproduction, in *Safety Evaluation of Drugs and Chemicals*, Lloyd, W. E., Ed., Hemisphere Publishing Corporation, Washington, 1986, chap. 13.

Manson, J. M. and Kang, Y. J. Test methods for assessing female reproductive and developmental toxicology, in *Principles and Methods in Toxicology*, Hayes, A. W., Ed., Raven Press, New York, 1982, chap. 11.

Manson, J. M. and Wise, L. D., Teratogens, in *Casarett and Doull's Toxicology*, Amdur, M. O., Doull, J., and Klaassen, C. D., Eds., Pergamon Press, New York, 1991, chap. 7.

Miller, R. K., Perinatal toxicology: its recognition and fundamentals, *Am. J. Indust. Med.*, 4, 205, 1983.

Miller, R. K., Kellogg, C. K., and Saltzman, R. A., Reproductive and perinatal toxicology, in *Handbook of Toxicology*, Haley, T. J. and Berndt, W. O., Eds., Hemisphere Publishing Corporation, Washington, 1987, chap. 7.

Murad, F. and Kuret, J. A., Estrogens and progestins, in *Goodman and Gilman's The Pharmacological Basis of Therapeutics*, Gilman, A. G., Rall, T. W., Nies, A. S., and Taylor, P., Eds., Pergamon Press, New York, 1990, chap. 58.

Radike, M., Reproductive toxicology, in *Industrial Toxicology*, Williams, P. L. and Burson, J. L., Eds., Van Nostrand Reinhold Company, New York, 1985, chap. 16.

Sipes, I. G. and Gandolfi, A. J., Biotransformation of toxicants, in *Casarett and Doull's Toxicology*, Amdur, M. O., Doull, J., and Klaassen, C. D., Eds., Pergamon Press, New York, 1991, chap. 4.

Thomas, J. A., Toxic responses of the reproductive system, in *Casarett and Doull's Toxicology*, Amdur, M. O., Doull, J., and Klaassen, C. D., Eds., Pergamon Press, New York, 1991, chap. 16.

Whorton, M. D., Bedinghaus, J., Obrinsky, D., and Spear, P. W., Reproductive disorders, in *Occupational Health*, Levy, B. S. and Wegman, D. H., Eds., Little, Brown, and Company, Boston, 1983, chap. 20.

Wilson, J. D., Androgens, in *Goodman and Gilman's The Pharmacological Basis of Therapeutics*, Gilman, A. G., Rall, T. W., Nies, A. S., and Taylor, P., Eds., Pergamon Press, New York, 1990, chap. 59.

Zenick, H. and Clegg, E. D., Assessment of male reproductive toxicity: a risk assessment approach, in *Principles and Methods in Toxicology*, Hayes, A. W., Ed., Raven Press, New York, 1982, chap. 10.

7   RESPIRATORY TOXICOLOGY

FUNCTION OF THE RESPIRATORY SYSTEM

The primary function of the respiratory system is to deliver oxygen to the bloodstream where it can be routed throughout the body to every cell, and to remove the waste product of metabolism—carbon dioxide. Cells require oxygen to carry out oxidative phosphorylation, the series of reactions whereby energy contained in chemical bonds in food is "repackaged" into the bonds in the molecule ATP (a form of energy the cell can directly use). Although some cells in the body can function without oxygen for a short time, many cells (such as heart cells or brain cells) are absolutely dependent on an adequate supply of oxygen in order to survive. The respiratory system also plays a role in the process of speech, the defense of the body, and the regulation of body pH. It is also a rapid route by which volatile xenobiotics can reach the brain.

ANATOMY AND PHYSIOLOGY OF THE RESPIRATORY SYSTEM

Respiratory Anatomy

The respiratory system can be divided into two basic parts (Figure 1). The first part, the *conducting portion*, is responsible for carrying air to and from the second part, *respiratory portion*. The respiratory portion is where the process of *gas exchange*, the movement of oxygen into and carbon dioxide out of the bloodstream occurs.

The conducting portion of the respiratory system begins with the *nose*. The external portion of the nose consists of cartilage covered with skin. The nostrils open into the internal portion of the nose, the *nasal cavity*, which is bounded below by the hard palate, and above and to the sides by other cranial bones. The nasal cavity is divided into halves by the nasal septum. Scroll-like bones called *conchae* project into the nasal cavity.

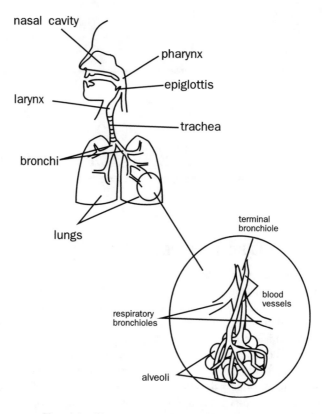

Figure 1   The anatomy of the respiratory system.

The nose is lined with epithelial tissue consisting of both column-shaped epithelial cells covered with cilia, and also cells called goblet cells that secrete mucus. Underneath the epithelial layer is a layer of connective tissue which contains many blood vessels. This combination of epithelium and connective tissue is called a *mucous membrane*.

The nose functions both to filter and to condition inhaled air. As air passes through the nose, entering particles become entrapped in the cilia and mucus. Also, the air is warmed and moistened as it passes over the warm, moist surfaces of the nasal mucous membranes. The nose also contains receptors for the sense of smell, and serves as a resonating chamber for the voice.

During inhalation, air moves from the nose into the *pharynx*. This chamber functions as a passageway between the nose and the larynx (which opens to the trachea) and also between the mouth and the esophagus (which leads to the stomach). The larynx is composed of cartilage lined with a mucous membrane. Folds of this membrane extend into the open center of the larynx, and vibrate as air passes over them. These are the *vocal cords*. Muscles in the larynx control the tension of the cords, as well as the size of the opening into the larynx, allowing the production of both high and low pitched sounds. A flexible flap called the *epiglottis* closes down over the top of the larynx during swallowing, preventing food or drink from entering the larynx. Irritation of the larynx produces a reflex action called a *cough*. In coughing, the opening to the larynx is temporarily closed, air is forced upward, pressure builds, and the larynx again opens to allow a blast of air out (hopefully taking with it any irritants). Severe irritation may even cause the larynx to clamp shut in a life-threatening spasm.

The larynx opens into the *trachea* or windpipe. This flexible tube is lined with mucous membrane, and is supported around the outside by C-shaped rings of cartilage. These rings keep the trachea from collapsing with the changes in air pressure which accompany breathing. At its base, the trachea branches into the *right and left primary bronchi* which lead to the right and left lungs. Within the lungs, the primary bronchi branch out into secondary bronchi, each of which leads to a different segment of the lung. Secondary bronchi continue to branch out, forming smaller tubules called *bronchioles*. The amount of cartilage in the airways decreases as the bronchi branch out and become smaller, until it finally disappears in the bronchioles. Smooth muscle content, however, increases, and bronchioles are completely ringed by a layer of smooth muscle. Spasms of that smooth muscle produce the condition called *asthma*.

Bronchioles continue to branch, forming *terminal bronchioles*, each of which branches into several *respiratory bronchioles*, which terminate in sacs called *alveoli*. The respiratory bronchioles and alveoli makeup the *respiratory portion* of the respiratory system—the area where gas exchange takes place. The extensive branching of bronchioles and expanded sacs

---

XENOBIOTIC METABOLISM
see also:
   Biotransformation   *Ch. 3, p. 21*

---

of the alveoli serves to dramatically increase surface area across which gas exchange occurs. Respiratory bronchioles and alveoli are made of one thin layer of epithelial tissue, with a thin layer of elastic fibers underneath. The epithelial tissue contains small cells called *Clara cells* (where xenobiotic metabolism may occur), thin flat *Type I cells*, and cuboidal *Type II* cells. Type II cells can divide to produce new Type I cells, and also can manufacture a substance called *surfactant*. Surfactant is a lipid-rich material that decreases surface tension in the alveoli, allowing the sacs to inflate properly and to remain inflated at expiration. *Alveolar macrophages*, cells that digest and destroy debris, are also found in the alveoli.

In order for gases to be exchanged between lungs and blood, there must be an adequate supply of blood in the area. The lungs are highly vascularized, with blood entering through the pulmonary arteries, which branch out into arterioles and finally capillaries. Networks of capillaries (which are made of one layer of thin, flat epithelial cells called *endothelium*) surround each terminal bronchiole and its respiratory bronchioles and alveoli. The capillaries then merge to form venules, which merge to form the pulmonary veins which carry oxygenated blood back to the heart.

Pulmonary Ventilation

The lungs are located in the thoracic cavity. A membrane called the *parietal pleura* covers the surface of each of the lungs and a membrane called the *visceral pleura* lines the walls of the thoracic cavity. The small space between these two membranes is called the *pleural cavity*, and is filled with fluid. The fluid acts as a lubricant, and also holds the two membrane surfaces together.

Breathing in, or *inspiration* is initiated by contraction of two muscles. As the *diaphragm*, a dome-shaped muscle that forms the floor of the thoracic cavity, contracts, it flattens out and increases the size of the thoracic cavity. At the same time, a set of muscles called the *external intercostals* contract, moving the ribs up and out, thereby also increasing the size of the thoracic cavity. As the thoracic cavity expands, the visceral pleura is pulled outward, pulling the parietal pleura outward, and expanding the volume of the lungs and inflating the alveoli. As the lung volume increases, pressure in the lung decreases, and air is pulled in through the conducting airways into the lung. A hole in the visceral or parietal pleura can allow air into the pleural cavity and break the seal between the membranes. This results in a *collapsed lung*, as pressure in the pleural cavity becomes greater than pressure in the lung.

Breathing out, or *expiration*, is usually a passive process, due to the elastic properties of the lungs. The muscles relax, and the volume of the thoracic cavity, and thus the lungs, decreases. When lung volume decreases, pressure in the lungs increases, and air is forced out of the lungs through the conducting airways.

Respiratory volumes can be measured using an instrument called a *spirometer*. The amount of air breathed in or out during normal quiet breathing is the *tidal volume* (TV). The additional volume of air that can be inhaled with effort is the *inspiratory reserve volume* (IRV). The additional volume of air that can be exhaled with effort is the *expiratory reserve volume* (ERV). TV + IRV + ERV together are called the *vital capacity*. No matter how hard you try, though, you can never expel all the air from of your lungs. The volume of air which always remains in your lungs is the *residual volume* (RV). Residual volume + vital capacity together make up the *total lung capacity*. The respiratory volumes are illustrated in Figure 2.

Respiratory rates can also be measured. The number of inspirations per minute is the *respiratory rate*. Respiratory rate multiplied by tidal volume gives the *minute volume*, the volume of air moved in and out per minute. Another common measurement is the FEV_1, the volume of air which can be forcibly exhaled in one second following maximum inhalation.

Many pathological conditions of the lungs affect respiratory volumes and rates. *Restrictive conditions* result from decrease in elasticity of the lungs, and

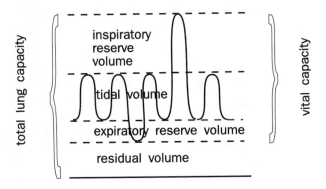

Figure 2   The respiratory volumes.

cause decreases in lung volumes. *Obstructive conditions* result from blockage or narrowing of the airways, and cause decreases in airflow rates, such as are measured by FEV_1.

Gas Exchange

In the respiratory bronchioles and alveoli, there are few barriers to the diffusion of gases. To move between alveoli and the bloodstream, gases need only cross a thin, flat Type I alveolar cell and a thin, flat capillary endothelial cell. The forces driving the diffusion of gases are the available surface area and the differences in concentration of the gas in alveoli, blood, and tissues. The concentration of a gas is reflected by its *partial pressure*, the pressure exerted by that particular gas in a given situation. For example, atmospheric pressure is the sum of all the partial pressures of the gases that makeup the atmosphere. Gases dissolved in liquids also have partial pressures. Gases tend to diffuse from areas of high partial pressure to areas of lower partial pressure.

Air which has just arrived in the alveoli has a relatively high partial pressure of oxygen, and a very low partial pressure of carbon dioxide. The partial pressure of oxygen in the bloodstream, however, is low, while the partial pressure of carbon dioxide is quite high. Thus, in the lungs, oxygen diffuses from the alveoli into the bloodstream, and carbon dioxide diffuses from the bloodstream into the alveoli. In the tissues, where oxygen is being consumed and carbon dioxide produced, oxygen partial pressure is low and carbon dioxide partial pressure is high. Blood traveling to the tissues, though, has just exited to the lungs and so has a high partial pressure of oxygen and a low partial pressure of carbon dioxide. Thus, in the tissues, oxygen leaves the bloodstream and diffuses into the tissues, while carbon dioxide leaves the tissues and diffuses into the bloodstream. Gas exchange in the lung is shown in Figure 3.

Most of the oxygen carried in the bloodstream, however, is not found dissolved in the blood fluid. Instead, it is carried by a special molecule called *hemo-*

HEMOGLOBIN
see also:
   Cardiovascular
     toxicology   *Ch. 8, p. 111*

globin, which is found in red blood cells. Hemoglobin will be discussed in Chapter 8. Most carbon dioxide is also carried in red blood cells. Some is bound to hemoglobin (at different sites than where oxygen is carried), but most combines with water to form *carbonic acid*, which then breaks down into a hydrogen ion and a bicarbonate ion. Bicarbonate ions then leave the red blood cells, and join with sodium in the plasma to make sodium bicarbonate. When carbon dioxide levels decline, the series of reactions runs in reverse to liberate carbon dioxide (Figure 4).

Control of Respiration

Rate and depth of respiration is controlled by the *respiratory centers*, located in an area of the brain called the brain stem. These centers control normal respiration, and also make the necessary responses to any changes in physiological status. Receptors located in the arteries monitor the partial pressures of both oxygen and carbon dioxide in the blood, and receptors in the brain monitor the partial pressure of carbon dioxide in cerebrospinal fluid. Actually, changes in carbon

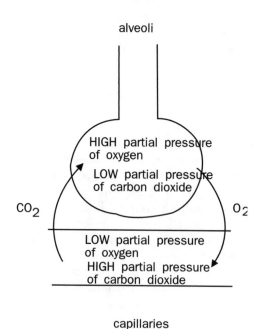

Figure 3 The process of gas exchange.

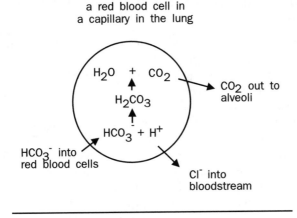

a red blood cell in
a capillary in the lung

H_2O + CO_2

CO_2 out to
alveoli

H_2CO_3

HCO_3^- + H^+

HCO_3^- into
red blood cells

Cl⁻ into
bloodstream

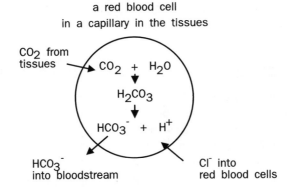

a red blood cell
in a capillary in the tissues

CO_2 from
tissues

CO_2 + H_2O

H_2CO_3

HCO_3^- + H^+

HCO_3^-
into bloodstream

Cl⁻ into
red blood cells

Figure 4 The carbon dioxide/carbonic acid/bicarbonate buffer system.

dioxide levels are not measured directly by these receptors—instead they respond to the accompanying changes in pH. (As carbon dioxide levels go up, carbonic acid levels go up, and hydrogen ion levels go up so pH goes down. Likewise, as carbon dioxide levels go down, carbonic acid levels go down, and hydrogen ion levels go down so pH goes up.)

It is changes in carbon dioxide levels which stimulate the greatest responses from the respiratory centers. If carbon dioxide levels go up, the rate of respiration is stimulated, leading to a more rapid release of carbon dioxide from the lungs. If carbon dioxide levels go down, rate of respiration is slowed.

Receptors also monitor expansion of the lungs, preventing overextension or collapse during forced inspiration and expiration. In addition, other receptors respond to changes in blood pressure, increasing rate of respiration when blood pressure goes down, and decreasing rate of respiration when blood pressure goes up.

EFFECTS OF TOXICANTS ON THE RESPIRATORY SYSTEM— GENERAL PRINCIPLES

Just as the respiratory system is an important route of exposure for various toxicants, it is also a target for many of them. For many toxicants, the lungs are a target only when the route of exposure to that toxicant is inhalation. Other toxicants, however, produce effects on the lungs even when exposures occur through ingestion or absorption through the skin.

Toxicants that affect the respiratory system following inhalation can be divided into two general categories: *gases* and *particulates*. The chemical and physical properties of these toxicants determine how they will be distributed in the respiratory system. Exposure to these toxicants can either be acute or chronic, and effects due to exposure may be either immediate or delayed. Of course, the respiratory system also has several defenses against injury by these toxicants. We will discuss defense mechanisms first, then the types of toxicants and their properties, then immediate effects, and then delayed effects. Finally, we will discuss laboratory testing of respiratory toxicants.

DEFENSE MECHANISMS OF THE RESPIRATORY SYSTEM

The respiratory system may be particularly vulnerable to exposure to toxicants, but it also has several defense mechanisms which help protect it. First of all, the cilia and mucus found in the mucous membranes of the upper airways help trap particles and prevent them from penetrating further into the lungs. Particles trapped in the mucus are moved along by motion of the cilia (in what has been termed the "*mucociliary escalator*") upward toward the mouth to be swallowed. Particles from the lower reaches of the lungs may be consumed by macrophages, which then move onto the mucociliary escalator for elimination. Particles may also leave the lungs through dissolution or absorption into the bloodstream or lymphatic system.

These clearance mechanisms may, however, be altered by exposure to toxicants. In heavy smokers, for example, rate of clearance of particles from the respiratory system is significantly slowed. This slowing might be due to inhibition of ciliary motion, changes in mucous viscosity, damage to macrophages, or a combination of factors. Damage to macrophages may not only slow clearance, but also lead to an increased risk of infection because macrophages are important in destruction of pathogens. An inherited disease which affects viscosity of mucus is *cystic fibrosis*. In cystic fibrosis, defects in chloride ion channels lead to the production of overly thick mucus which blocks the airways and shuts down the mucociliary escalator, leading to difficulties with ventilation complicated by frequent infections. Other organs, such as those of the digestive system, are frequently affected in cystic fibrosis as well.

There are also many cells of the immune system located within the lungs, ready to respond to invaders. Some of these cells produce antibodies against foreign antigens, and others release endogenous chemicals which mediate allergic

responses (such as symptoms of
asthma or bronchitis). Thus, as
well as being protective, the
presence of these cells means
that exposure to some toxicants
can trigger an allergic attack or
chronic inflammation.

| IMMUNE SYSTEM |
| see also: |
| Immunotoxicology   Ch. 12, p. 171 |

If, in spite of other defense mechanisms, damage to alveolar cells occurs,
some repair is possible. When Type I cells are damaged, Type II cells undergo
mitosis, proliferate, and replace the damaged cells. And, remember, Clara cells
also contain cytochrome P450 and are capable of carrying out xenobiotic
metabolism.

TYPES OF RESPIRATORY TOXICANTS

Gases and particles suspended in gases can be inhaled easily. Because the
amount of a gas or particle which is inhaled and retained is difficult to measure
exactly, exposures can be estimated based on the concentration of the gas or particle in the environment and the length of exposure. Of course other factors, such
as breathing rate and depth, also can influence exposure.

Typically, concentration of gases are expressed as *parts per million* or *ppm*.
This unit expresses concentration as the volume of the gas per million volumes of
air. Concentrations of gases and suspended particles as well may also be
expressed in a weight per volume manner, usually as *milligrams per cubic meter
of air (mg/m^3)*.

Based on laboratory and epidemiological studies, the American Conference
of Governmental and Industrial Hygienists has developed a list of allowable
exposures in the occupational setting to various respiratory toxicants. These
Threshold Limit Values (TLVs) specify the average maximum allowable concentrations to which workers can be exposed without undue risk. The TLV-TWA
(time-weighted average) gives the maximum allowable concentration for exposure averaged over an 8-hour day. The TLV-STEL (short-term exposure limit)
gives the maximum allowable concentration for a 15-min period, and the TLV-C
(ceiling) gives the concentration limit that should never be exceeded. Some representative TLVs are shown in Table 1.

Gases

Deposition of a gas in the respiratory system depends primarily on the water
solubility of the gas. Water soluble gases are likely to dissolve into the watery
mucus secreted by the cells lining the upper parts of the respiratory tract. Gases
which are less water soluble are more likely to continue deeper into the respiratory tract.

**TABLE 1   Examples of some threshold limit
values (TLVs)**

Substance	TLV-TWA (ppm)	TLV-STEL (ppm)
Ammonia	25	35
Benzene	10	30
Ethyl ether	400	1200
Ozone	0.1	0.2
Trichloroethylene	100	535

Particulates

For particulates, size is the main factor that influences deposition in the respiratory system. Very large particles (greater than 5 µm in diameter) are likely to impact on the walls of the nasal cavity or pharynx during inspiration. Medium-sized particles (1 to 5 µm in diameter) tend to sediment (settle) out in the trachea, bronchi, or bronchioles as air velocity decreases in these smaller passageways. Particles less than 1 µm in diameter typically move by diffusion into alveoli.

Physiologic factors may influence particle deposition as well. The narrower the airways, the more deposition that will occur. Rapid inhalation of deep breaths (such as may occur during exercise) also increases exposure and deposition.

IMMEDIATE RESPONSES TO RESPIRATORY TOXICANTS

Many gases and particulates are *irritants*, and produce their effects within a few minutes to a few hours following exposure. Injury to the epithelial cells lining the respiratory tract can produce an inflammatory response, characterized by increase in permeability of blood vessels and accumulation of immune system cells in the area of the damage. Cell death, or *necrosis*, may also result.

The increase in blood vessel permeability leads to an accumulation of fluids, or *edema* in the airways. Exposure to water soluble irritants such as *sulfur dioxide* (SO_2) produces swelling and edema in the upper airways, causing narrowing of the passageways, and making breathing more difficult. Irritation may also produce an increase in secretion of mucus. Studies have shown that exposure to as little as 5 ppm sulfur dioxide can affect airways. *Formaldehyde* is another upper airway irritant.

SULFUR DIOXIDE
see also:

   Air pollution   **Ch. 14, p. 204**
   Sulfur dioxide   **Appendix, p. 246**

FORMALDEHYDE
see also:

   Immunotoxicology   **Ch. 12, p. 177**
   Air pollution   **Ch. 14, p. 206**
   Formaldehyde   **Appendix, p. 238**

Exposure to irritants can also promote contraction of the ring of smooth muscle surrounding bronchioles, an effect known as *bronchoconstriction*. This can happen either by direct action of the irritant itself, or through an irritant-produced increase in sensitivity of bronchiolar smooth muscle to other agents (other irritants, or perhaps even endogenous substances). Sulfur dioxide is also a potent bronchoconstrictor. Individuals with preexisting respiratory diseases such as asthma may be particularly susceptible. Some of the same effects (swelling and bronchoconstriction) can also be produced by agents which are not direct irritants, but instead may produce an allergic response.

Accumulation of fluid in the alveoli interferes with gas exchange, with the fluid acting as an additional barrier to diffusion. Irritant gases and particles which are less water soluble, such as *nitrogen dioxide* (NO_2) and *ozone* (O_3) produce these effects. Exposure of rats to as little as 1 ppm ozone has caused cell death and edema. Ozone, an oxidant, may damage membranes or inhibit enzymes within the cells, probably through the process of lipid peroxidation. Although relatively insoluble in water, nitrogen dioxide is slightly absorbed all along the respiratory tract, producing both upper and lower airway irritation. Like ozone, nitrogen dioxide is also an oxidant.

NITROGEN DIOXIDE
see also:
  Air pollution   *Ch. 14, p. 204*
  Nitrogen dioxide   *Appendix, p. 240*

OZONE
see also:
  Air pollution   *Ch. 14, p. 206*
  Ozone   *Appendix, p. 242*

One very unique respiratory toxicant is the herbicide paraquat. With an LD_{50} of 30 mg/kg, it is quite toxic. What is unique about paraquat is that it accumulates in and damages the lungs no matter what the route of absorption: respiratory, oral, or dermal. Paraquat seems to accumulate in Type II cells by an active transport process. Paraquat, too, may produce damage through lipid peroxidation, although the mechanism of action is not completely clear.

PARAQUAT
see also:
  Water pollution   *Ch. 15, p. 210*
  Paraquat   *Appendix, p. 243*

DELAYED AND CUMULATIVE RESPONSES TO RESPIRATORY TOXICANTS

Repeated (chronic) exposure to respiratory toxicants often leads to long-term changes in respiratory function, some of which may not occur until some time after exposure to the toxicant begins, and others which may accumulate gradually before noticeable changes occur. These changes may lead to obstructive or restrictive lung diseases or lung cancer, and are typically irreversible.

TOLUENE DIISOCYANATE (TDI)
see also:
Immunotoxicology   *Ch. 12, p. 176*
TDI   *Appendix, p. 247*

Asthma is an acute effect to which a chronic predisposition may develop following exposure to toxicants. For example, exposure to the chemical toluene diisocyanate (TDI) can lead to development of asthma. Not only do individuals with TDI-induced asthma react to even very low levels of TDI, but many also suffer the generalized increase in sensitivity of airway smooth muscle mentioned earlier. Exposure to cotton dust can produce a condition called *byssinosis* (also sometimes called "brown lung") which is also characterized by bronchoconstriction. Symptoms of byssinosis seems to be most severe when a worker in a cotton mill returns to work after a day or two off. For this reason it is also termed "Monday morning sickness." The cause of byssinosis is not clear—it may be an allergic reaction to microorganisms on the dust particles, or a simple reaction to an irritant in the cotton dust itself.

Another type of allergic reaction is *hypersensitivity pneumonitis*. Symptoms of this problem are shortness of breath, fever, and chills. Hypersensitivity pneumonitis results from exposure to organic materials which trigger an immune response localized primarily in the lower airways. Exposure to moldy hay, for example, can lead to a condition called Farmer's Lung, while exposure to fungus found on cheese particles may produce Cheese Washer's Lung. Continued exposure can result in permanent lung damage in the form of fibrosis (see below).

Chronic bronchitis is another obstructive condition which may be related to toxicant exposure. In bronchitis, excessive secretion of mucus causes a chronic cough. Both smoking and exposure to high levels of air pollution seem to be risk factors in the development of chronic bronchitis. The risk of developing *emphysema*, an obstructive disease characterized by breakdown of walls of alveoli and loss of elasticity, is also high for smokers.

A number of different toxicants which produce irritation and inflammation in the lower respiratory system may, after some years of exposure, lead to a restrictive condition called *fibrosis*. Fibrosis occurs when repeated activation of macrophages leads to chronic inflammation of an area. This results in the recruitment of *fibroblasts*, cells which proliferate and produce the rigid protein *collagen*. The accumulation of collagen interferes with ventilation (by reducing elasticity) and blood flow within the lung.

Toxicants which produce fibrosis include crystalline silicates. In *silicosis*, one of the most widespread and serious occupational lung diseases, macrophages try to ingest the silica crystals, and are destroyed in the attempt. This results in the release of digestive enzymes, and the rerelease of the silica which is then available for ingestion by other macrophages. Silica crystals thus accumulate in the lungs, surrounded by areas of inflammation. Fibroblasts then proliferate, and produce the collagen nodules which characterize this disease.

Asbestosis, a similar condition, is caused by exposure to asbestos, itself a fibrous silicate. There are several different forms of asbestos, including serpentine forms (a group to which the most commonly used type, chrysotile asbestos, belongs) and amphibole forms. From the 1940s to the 1960s a significant number of workers were exposed to asbestos, and later developed asbestosis. Exposure to asbestos is also linked to development of

ASBESTOS
see also:
  Asbestos   *Appendix, p. 234*

CANCER
see also:
  Carcinogenesis   *Ch. 5, p. 55*

not only the more common form of lung cancer (tumors originating in lung epithelial cells) but also of a relatively rare form of cancer called *mesothelioma*. There can be an extremely long latent period (as much as 40 years) between exposure to asbestos and development of mesothelioma.

Currently, concern over asbestos focuses on whether or not there are significant risks associated with exposure of the general public to fibers which may be shed from asbestos-containing products such as insulation, brake linings, etc. There is considerable debate in the research community, as well, over whether the different forms of asbestos are equally dangerous. The answers to these questions will prove significant as decisions are made on whether or not to attempt to remove existing asbestos in buildings (an expensive and difficult process).

Of course one of the greatest risk factors for lung cancer is exposure to tobacco smoke. It has been well established that smokers have a 10 to 20 times greater risk of developing lung cancer than nonsmokers, and that

SMOKING
see also:
  Tobacco   *Appendix, p. 247*

smoking interacts in an additive or in some cases synergistic manner with other risk factors for lung cancer (such as asbestos). Lately, research has focused on the risks of *"second-hand" cigarette smoke* to nonsmokers. Sidestream smoke (from the end of the cigarette) makes up a significant amount of second-hand smoke, and may have even higher concentrations of toxicants than inhaled smoke, as well as smaller average particle size. Studies have shown that children and nonsmoking spouses of smokers are more likely to suffer from respiratory problems and lung cancer, respectively, than children and spouses of nonsmokers.

One other well-known occupational lung disease is "black lung"—*coal worker's pneumoconiosis* or *CWP*. Caused by exposure to coal dust, CWP is characterized by the presence in the lungs of black nodules, along with widespread fibrosis and emphysema. Also, American veterans of the war in Kuwait and Iraq are being examined after complaining of delayed illness following inhalation of smoke from massive petroleum fires.

INHALATION STUDIES

In the laboratory, toxicologists use inhalation chambers to study effects of airborne toxicants. An inhalation chamber consists of one or more areas in which animals are held for exposure, along with some apparatus for delivery of the toxicant to be tested. In *static test systems*, the toxicant is simply introduced and mixed into the atmosphere in a closed chamber. Although this method is relatively simple, disadvantages include the tendency for oxygen to be depleted and carbon dioxide to accumulate in the chamber, and the constantly decreasing concentration of the toxicant in the atmosphere as it settles out or is absorbed. One way around these difficulties is to use a *dynamic test system*. In this system, air is constantly circulated through the exposure chamber, with the toxicant being introduced into the entering airstream. Gases may be directly mixed in with incoming air; particles may be introduced either as a dry dust or suspended in droplets of water. Concentration of gases, and concentration and size of particles can be monitored by sampling within the chamber, and level of exposure can be adjusted by altering either flow rate through the chamber or rate of addition of the toxicant to the airstream.

The chambers in which the animals are exposed may vary also. The whole body of the animal may be exposed to the toxicant, or just the head or neck. In the latter systems, restraint of the animal may pose a problem, but the problems of deposition of toxicant on the animal's coat and subsequent ingestion by licking are solved. Also, if the chamber containing the body can be sealed, it can be adapted as a *plethysmograph*, so that pressure changes within the chamber can be used to estimate lung volumes. Toxicants may also be injected directly into the trachea.

Along with measuring respiratory rates and volumes (vital capacity, minute volume, FEV_1, etc.), other parameters such as oxygen and carbon dioxide levels, and blood pH can also be used to assess respiratory function in test animals. In addition to *in vivo* studies, washing of the lungs with physiological saline (a technique called *bronchoalveolar lavage*) can supply cells for *in vitro* analysis of cellular function. This technique is particularly useful for studying macrophages.

REFERENCES

Duffell, G. M., Pulmonotoxicity: toxic effects in the lung, in *Industrial Toxicology*, Williams, P. L. and Burson, J. L., Eds., Van Nostrand Reinhold, New York, 1985, chap. 9.

Gordon, T. and Amdur, M. O., Responses of the respiratory system to toxic agents, in *Casarett and Doull's Toxicology*, Amdur, M. O., Doull, J., and Klaassen, C. D., Eds., Pergamon Press, New York, 1991, chap. 12.

Horton, A. A. and Fairhurst, S., Lipid peroxidation and mechanisms of toxicity, *CRC Crit. Rev. Toxicol.*, 18, 27, 1987.

Kennedy, G. L., Jr., Inhalation toxicology, in *Principles and Methods of Toxicology*, Hayes, A. W., Ed., Raven Press, New York, 1989, chap. 12.

Marshall, E., Involuntary smokers face health risks, *Science*, 234, 1066, 1986.

McClellan, R. O. and Hobbs, C. H., Generation, characterization, and exposure systems for test atmospheres, in *Safety Evaluation of Drugs and Chemicals*, Lloyd, W. E., Ed., Hemisphere, Washington, 1986, chap. 17.

National Safety Council, Olishifski, J. B., Ed., *Fundamentals of Industrial Hygiene*, 2nd ed., National Safety Council, Chicago, 1983.

Reasor, M. J., The composition and dynamics of environmental tobacco smoke, *J. Environ. Health*, 50, 20, 1987.

Stone, R., No meeting of the minds on asbestos, *Science*, 254, 928, 1991.

Wegman, D. H., Respiratory disorders, in *Occupational Health*, Levy, B. S. and Wegman, D. H., Eds., Little, Brown, and Company, Boston, 1983, chap. 18.

Witschi, H. and Last, J. A., Pulmonary toxicology, in *Handbook of Toxicology*, Haley, T. J. and Berndt, W. O. Eds., Hemisphere, Washington, 1987, chap. 5.

8

CARDIOVASCULAR TOXICOLOGY

FUNCTION OF THE CARDIOVASCULAR SYSTEM

The basic function of the cardiovascular system is transport. It is responsible for carrying gases, nutrients, waste products, cells, and other substances from one part of the body to another. It consists of a pump (the heart), a network of tubes (the vascular system), and a transport fluid (the blood). All three components can be affected by toxicants.

ANATOMY AND PHYSIOLOGY OF THE HEART

The heart (Figure 1) is a hollow muscular organ located in the thoracic cavity. The bulk of the heart, the *myocardium*, is composed of cardiac muscle tissue. The outside of the heart is covered by a connective tissue sac called the *pericardium*, while the inside of the heart is lined by a layer of epithelial and connective tissue called the *endocardium*. The heart contains four *chambers*: the *right atrium*, the *right ventricle*, the *left atrium*, and the *left ventricle*. The right and left sides of the heart are separated by a wall of tissue called a *septum*.

Blood which is low in oxygen and high in carbon dioxide enters the heart from the *inferior vena cava* and *superior vena cava*—the two major veins which collect blood from all body tissues. This deoxygenated blood enters into the right atrium, and then passes through the *tricuspid valve* (a one-way structure which prevents backflow of blood into the atrium) into the right ventricle. From the right ventricle, the blood is pumped through the *pulmonary semilunar valve* into the *pulmonary arteries*, which carry blood to the lungs to replenish oxygen and release carbon dioxide. The oxygenated blood returns to the heart from the lungs through the *pulmonary veins*, which empty into the left atrium. Blood passes from the left atrium through the *bicuspid (mitral) valve* and into the left ventricle. From here the oxygenated blood is pumped through the *aortic semilunar valve* into the *aorta*, through which it is distributed to the rest of the body.

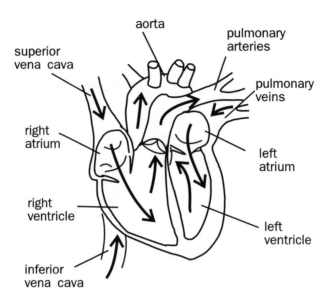

Figure 1 A coronal section through the heart.

The force required to move blood through these pathways is supplied by the beating action of the heart. During a single heartbeat or *cardiac cycle*, the atria contract together, pushing blood into the ventricles, then the atria relax while the ventricles contract and push blood to the lungs and the rest of the body.

Contraction of the various chambers are produced by the synchronized contraction of cardiac muscle fibers, which are joined together at special communicating junctions called *intercalated discs*. The basis for excitability of cardiac cells lies in the distribution of ions across their membrane. At rest, the interior of a cardiac cell is about 80 to 90 mV more negative than the exterior. This difference is called a *membrane potential*. A membrane pump (the Na$^+$/K$^+$ ATPase) maintains a gradient with a high concentration of sodium outside the cell, and a high concentration of potassium within the cell. Small shifts in ionic currents cause a gradual *depolarization* (in other words, the membrane potential becomes less negative) and eventually a threshold is reached. At this threshold, sodium channels in the membrane open, allowing sodium to rush into the cell, and altering the membrane potential from negative to positive. At this point, the sodium channels close, and other ion channels open, including a calcium channel. (Influx of calcium ions, along with release of intercellular calcium, triggers contraction of the muscle fiber.) Finally, potassium channels open allowing an outward movement of potassium. This returns the membrane potential to the original negative potential (a process called *repolarization*). The action of the Na$^+$/K$^+$ ATPase, of course, rapidly rebuilds the original gradient. This process is shown in Figure 2.

The excitatory impulse passes from one cardiac muscle cell to the next through the intercalated disks. The time between the passage of one impulse until

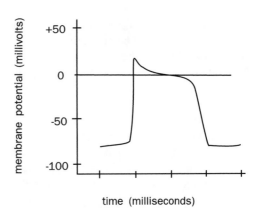

Figure 2
Changes in membrane potential in a
cardiac muscle cell during depolarization.

the muscle cell is ready to respond to the next impulse is called the *refractory period.*

Many heart muscle cells can contract spontaneously (a property known as *automaticity*). Cells showing automaticity undergo spontaneous depolarization caused primarily by an inward sodium current.

Rates of contraction are normally controlled by a group of cells in the upper part of the right atrium called the *sinoatrial (SA) node.* These cells have the most rapid rate of spontaneous depolarization and thus initiate an impulse before other cells have a chance to. Impulses from these "pacemaker" cells spread rapidly throughout the atria (causing them to contract simultaneously) and eventually reach a second group of specialized cells in the lower part of the right atrium called the *atrioventricular (AV) node.* Here the impulse is delayed briefly, then is sent down a bundle of fibers which run down the septum between the two ventricles. From this bundle, fibers called *Purkinje fibers* spread out, carrying the impulse to contract to all ventricular muscle cells. The electrical activity of the heart may be viewed on an *electrocardiogram.*

The SA node controls heart rate through its own spontaneous automaticity, but the rate of depolarization can be affected by the autonomic nervous system. Stimulation of the sympathetic nervous system causes an increase in heart rate, while stimulation of the parasympathetic nervous system causes a decrease in heart rate.

EFFECTS OF TOXICANTS ON THE HEART

Arrhythmias

One way in which toxicants can interfere with cardiovascular function is through interference with the electrochemical system which regulates contraction of the heart. Abnormalities in this system lead to irregularities in heartbeat, or *arrhythmias*. There are many different types of arrhythmias, with perhaps the most serious being completely asynchronous contraction of muscle cells, or *fibrillation*. Because the ventricles must pump blood with so much more force than the atria (which for the most part empty almost passively into the ventricles), ventricular arrhythmias are typically much more serious than atrial arrhythmias.

Arrhythmias can be produced through effects on the SA node. Excessive sympathetic stimulation can lead to rapid heartbeat (*tachycardia*) while excessive parasympathetic stimulation can lead to a slowed heartbeat (*bradycardia*). Thus, cardiovascular effects can be produced indirectly by toxicants that affect the autonomic nervous system. Damage to cells of the SA node can also produce arrhythmias by interfering with their automaticity. (Often, if SA node cells are unable to perform, cells of the AV node will attempt to compensate, setting the rhythm of the heart.) *Halogenated hydrocarbons* (chloro- and fluorocarbons) are one class of compounds which alter activity of the SA node. These compounds suppress activity of the SA node cells, and at the same time reduce the refractory period of Purkinje cells. This makes the ventricles in particular more sensitive to the effects of catecholamines (the neurotransmitters released by the sympathetic nervous system) thus increasing the ability of sympathetic stimulation to produce tachycardia and arrhythmias.

HALOGENATED HYDROCARBON SOLVENTS
see also:

Alterations in automaticity may occur in other cells as well, frequently through effects on ion channels. Sometimes, cells in the Purkinje network, or even normal atrial or ventricular cells may spontaneously depolarize, producing extra, or *ectopic* beats. Some toxicants such as the alkaloid *aconitine* (found in the plant monkshood) keep sodium channels open, preventing repolarization and leading to the repeated generation of impulses.

In other cases, impulse generation may be inhibited by toxicants. For example, drugs including the *tricyclic antidepressants* suppress activity in Purkinje cells, probably through blockade of sodium channels. This leads to an increase in duration of impulses and increase in

---

TTX, STX
see also:

---

the refractory period, thus delaying conduction to the ventricles. At high enough exposures, complete blocks may result (particularly in the AV node where blocks are most common). Other sodium channel blockers such as the biological toxins *tetrodotoxin* and *saxitoxin* have similar effects; however, nervous system effects usually overshadow the cardiovascular effects.

Direct, immediate damage to cardiac muscle cells, or *myocarditis*, can also cause arrhythmias, delays, or blocks in the passage of impulses. Myocarditis can result from direct action of toxicants or can be due to inflammation resulting from hypersensitivity (allergic) reactions to drugs such as penicillin.

Cardiomyopathies and Other Effects on Cardiac Muscle

Contractility, the ability of cardiac muscle to contract, can also be affected by toxicants. Decreases in contractility lead to congestive heart failure, a condition in which the heart is unable to pump sufficiently to supply blood to all tissues. Individuals with congestive heart failure may suffer from fatigue and edema (accumulation of fluid in tissues) as well as hypertrophy of heart muscle. Decreases in contractility can result from toxicant-induced damage to cardiac muscle cells as well as other factors such as disruption of oxygen supply.

Gradual damage to cardiac muscle cells occurring over an extended period of time is called *cardiomyopathy*. Exposure to *cobalt*, a heavy metal which may block calcium channels, can lead to cardiomyopathy. Although problems with exposure to cobalt occur primarily in the workplace, the association between cobalt and heart disease was first noted in individuals who consumed beer containing 1 ppm cobalt as a foam-stabilizing agent. Some drugs, including the anti-tumor drug daunorubicin also produce cardiomyopathy. In this case, the mechanism of action is possibly related to the drug's apparent ability to bind to and damage nucleic acids.

Other agents which diminish the availability of calcium (such as other heavy metals including lead or cadmium) can also produce decreases in contractility. The drug *digitalis* (which is derived from the foxglove plant), on the other hand, enhances contractility through increasing calcium levels inside cardiac muscle cells. Digitalis inhibits the Na^+/K^+ ATPase, leading to increased levels of sodium within the cell. This sodium is then available to participate in an Na^+/Ca^{++} exchange mechanism. These changes can, however, also lead to arrhythmias.

THE VASCULAR SYSTEM

The heart pumps blood through a network of vessels called the vascular system (Figure 3). *Arteries*, the vessels which carry blood away from the heart, are generally large elastic vessels. They consist of an inner layer of epithelial cells and connective tissue (containing many elastic fibers) called the *endothelium*, a middle layer of smooth muscle, and an outer connective tissue covering. As dis-

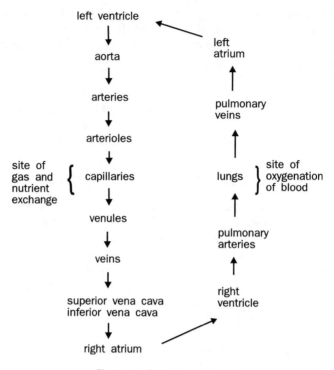

Figure 3   The vascular system.

tance from the heart increases, arteries branch and decrease in size. Other changes occur also, with the relative amount of elastic fibers decreasing and the relative amount of smooth muscle increasing. Eventually, arteries become *arterioles*, which are much smaller vessels made only of the endothelial layer and a few smooth muscle cells. Arterioles branch into capillaries, which consist of simply an endothelial layer. The endothelium of capillaries may be continuous, or it may have pores or gaps. Capillaries are the site of the highest ratio of surface area to mass of a tissue, and are where gas and material exchange between the blood and the tissues occurs.

At the junction between arterioles and capillaries, there is a band of smooth muscle. This *sphincter* regulates blood flow in the capillary by contracting (shutting off blood flow) and relaxing (allowing blood flow). Additional methods of regulation of blood flow include contraction of smooth muscle in arterioles, and routing of blood through vessels called *anastomoses* which supply a direct connection between arterioles and venules and bypass capillaries.

To return blood to the heart, capillaries merge to form *venules*, which in turn merge to form *veins*. Veins have much thinner, less muscular walls than arteries. Veins also have valves to prevent backflow of blood (these are necessary because the blood pressure which keeps blood moving in arteries drops very low in veins).

There are two primary circulation systems in the body. In the *pulmonary circuit*, blood leaves the right ventricle of the heart through the pulmonary arteries, which carry blood to the lungs for oxygenation. Oxygenated blood returns from the lungs through the *pulmonary veins*, and enters the left atrium. In the *systemic circuit*, blood from the left ventricle leaves the heart through the *aorta*, and is distributed throughout the body. A few of the major arteries include the *carotid arteries* which supply the head and neck region (including the brain), the *coronary arteries* which supply the heart itself, the *subclavian arteries* which supply the chest, shoulders, and arms, the *celiac* and *mesenteric arteries* which supply the gastrointestinal organs, the *renal arteries* which supply the kidneys, and the *iliac arteries* which supply the pelvic region and legs. After passing through the capillary network, blood then returns to the heart through the veins. The *jugular vein* (which drains the head and neck region) as well as other veins from the upper part of the body merge to form the *superior vena cava* and the *hepatic* (from the liver), *renal* (from the kidneys), and other veins from the lower part of the body merge to form the *inferior vena cava*. The superior vena cava and inferior vena cava then flow into the right atrium.

EFFECTS OF TOXICANTS ON THE VASCULAR SYSTEM

Atherosclerosis

Atherosclerosis is a condition characterized by accumulation of *plaques*, lipid-containing masses which can form in the lumen of blood vessels and can severely narrow them (Figure 4). This of course restricts blood flow, and if a blood clot forms or becomes lodged at a plaque, blood flow may be completely blocked. This is particularly damaging if it occurs in arteries which supply tissues that depend heavily on a constant supply of oxygen. For example, blockage in cerebral vessels leads to death of brain tissue and is termed a *cerebrovascular accident* (or "stroke"). Blockage of coronary vessels leads to death of cardiac tissue and is termed a *myocardial infarction* (or "heart attack").

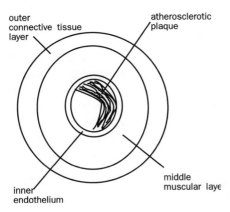

Figure 4
The process of athersclerosis.

The process by which plaques form is not completely understood, but probably involves damage to endothelial cells, proliferation of smooth muscle, invasion of the area by immune system cells, adhesion of platelets, and accumulation of lipids by the cells involved. Risk factors for development of atherosclerosis include high levels of blood cholesterol (which results from a combination of genetic factors and diet), high blood pressure, age (it is more common in older than in younger individuals), and sex (it is more common in men than in women, but the risk factor for women rises at menopause).

Toxicant exposure has also been implicated in some cases of atherosclerosis. Exposure to *carbon disulfide* has been reported in both laboratory and epidemiological studies to produce a significant increase in incidence of atherosclerosis. Carbon disulfide may initiate or accelerate the atherosclerotic process by direct injury to endothelial cells, by alterations in metabolism which increase cholesterol levels, or by a combination of these mechanisms. Chronic exposure to *carbon monoxide* also appears to accelerate the production of atherosclerotic plaques. It is unclear whether this is a direct effect on the vessels, or a by-product of CO-induced hypoxia (lack of sufficient oxygen). In either case, the carbon monoxide found in cigarette smoke may be one factor behind the observation that smokers are at higher risk for atherosclerosis than nonsmokers.

CARBON DISULFIDE
see also:
Neurotoxicology ***Ch. 9. p. 138***
Carbon disulfide ***Appendix, p. 235***

CARBON MONOXIDE
see also:
Cellular sites of action ***Ch. 4, p. 49***
Cardiovascular toxicology ***Ch. 8, p. 114***
Air pollution ***Ch. 14, p. 202***
Carbon monoxide ***Appendix, p. 236***

Vascular Spasms and Blood Pressure

Some substances can affect vascular smooth muscle, produce changes in muscle tone, and thus change blood flow to an area of tissue. Endogenous compounds such as catecholamines interact with a type of receptor called an α-adrenergic receptor on vascular smooth muscle to produce vasoconstriction. Widespread vasoconstriction increases the resistance to blood flow, and thus blood pressure generally must rise in order to maintain adequate flow. Many drugs used to treat high blood pressure block catecholamine action by blocking alpha-adrenergic receptors.

An example of a toxicant that affects vascular smooth muscle is a class of compounds called *nitrates*. Nitrates and related compounds (probably through formation of nitric oxide) acti-vate an enzyme called guanylate cyclase which interacts with other enzymes to produce relax-ation of the smooth muscle. This vasodilation is one of the ways in which the drug nitroglycerin reduces heart pain (*angina*) which is caused by reduced

---

NITRATES
see also:

Cellular sites	*Ch. 4, p. 50*
Cardiovascular toxic	*Ch. 8, p. 115*
Water pollution	*Ch. 15, p. 221*
Nitrates	*Appendix, p. 240*

---

blood flow to cardiac tissue. Exposure to nitrates may occur in the explosives or pharmaceutical industries, and can produce headache (caused by dilation of cere-bral blood vessels) or dizziness (caused by reduced blood pressure). After a period of time, however, a tolerance to the nitrates may develop, and symptoms may disappear. At this point, however, cessation of exposure may trigger reflex-ive vasospasms, and sudden death from myocardial infarction may occur.

Hypertension, or high blood pressure, is a complex condition which is not well understood, but evidence has accumulated that chronic exposure to toxi-cants may play a role in some cases. *Cadmium*, for example, has produced hypertension in rats at levels of 5 ppm in drink-ing water, and exposure to lead also may be a risk factor for hypertension.

CADMIUM
see also:

Reproductive	
toxicology	*Ch. 6, p. 75*
Renal toxicology	*Ch. 11, p. 165*
Water pollution	*Ch. 15, p. 222*
Cadmium	*Appendix, p. 235*

THE BLOOD

Blood consists of a liquid called *plasma*, and a variety of cells including *red blood cells, white blood cells*, and cell fragments called *platelets*. Plasma is mostly water, but also contains dissolved salts, nutrients, gases, and plasma pro-teins such as *albumins* which are transport proteins, *globulins* which have roles in transport and immune function, and *fibrinogen*, a soluble protein which is con-verted to the insoluble fibrin during the blood clotting process.

Red blood cells, or erythrocytes, are biconcave disks with no nuclei. Proteins on the surface of red blood cells determine a person's blood type. Red blood cells contain the oxygen-carrying molecule *hemoglobin* (Figure 5). Hemoglobin is a protein composed of four subunits, each of which contains a heme molecule (a porphyrin ring containing an iron atom). Each heme molecule is capable of com-bining with one molecule of oxygen (O_2). A number of factors influence the bind-ing of oxygen to hemoglobin. When partial pressure of oxygen is low, cells

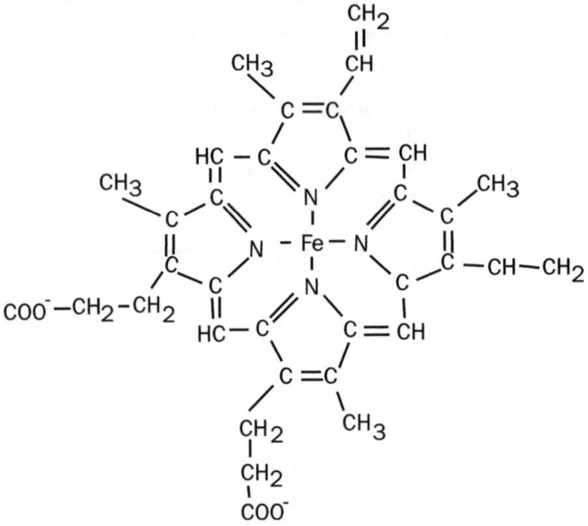

Figure 5 The structure of hemoglobin: a heme unit.

produce a molecule called 2,3-diphosphoglycerate which interacts with hemoglobin to encourage release of oxygen. Other factors that enhance oxygen release
include low blood pH (a reflection of higher carbon dioxide levels) and higher
temperatures. Higher blood pH (a reflection of lower carbon dioxide levels), and
lower temperatures, on the other hand, enhances binding of oxygen to hemoglobin. A phenomenon called *cooperativity* also exists. The four heme subunits
"cooperate" together in that release of one oxygen molecule alters the conformation of the hemoglobin molecule, and facilitates release of the other oxygens.
Likewise, binding of one oxygen molecule facilitates binding of others.

Red blood cells have a lifetime of about 120 days. They are produced in the
bone marrow in a process stimulated by a hormone called erythropoietin (made by
the kidneys) which is released in response to oxygen deficiency. Production also
requires sufficient quantities of vitamin B_{12}, folic acid, and iron, which is also partially recycled from red cells which are destroyed.

There are five types of white blood cells, or leukocytes normally found in the
blood. *Neutrophils*, *eosinophils*, and *basophils* are characterized by the presence
of granules in their cytoplasm. Neutrophils carry out phagocytosis, eosinophils
help regulate and control allergic reactions, while basophils release histamine and
other mediators of allergic reactions. *Monocytes* and *lymphocytes*, on the other
hand, lack granules. Monocytes leave the bloodstream and upon entering tissues
become macrophages—cells which are also important in phagocytosis.
Lymphocytes are involved in the production of specific immune responses,
responses which are directed against a specific invader (more about this in
Chapter 12).

Platelets are cell fragments which are involved in the process of *hemostasis* (cessation of blood loss). When a blood vessel is damaged, smooth muscle fibers near the injury contract (slowing blood loss from the damaged area), platelets adhere to the damaged endothelium, and clotting factors initiate the conversion of the soluble protein fibrinogen into the insoluble fibrin. More platelets stick to the strands of fibrin, and the clot draws the edges of the damaged area together. After repair occurs, the clot dissolves.

EFFECTS OF TOXICANTS ON THE BLOOD

Anemias, Hemolysis, and Related Disorders

One site at which chemicals can interfere with functioning of the blood is the bone marrow. Damage to bone marrow can lead to *pancytopenia*, a decrease in the numbers of red and white cells and platelets. Severe damage or outright destruction prevents stem cells from producing any new cells, a condition called *aplastic anemia*. Toxicants which can cause pancytopenia and/or aplastic anemia include drugs such as *chloramphenicol*, an antibiotic; *lindane*, an insecticide which is a chlorinated cyclohexane derived from benzene; and *benzene* itself. Chronic exposure to benzene levels of 100 ppm or higher can produce either a reversible pancytopenia or the more severe aplastic anemia. Benzene exposure has also

BENZENE
see also:
  Immunotoxicology   *Ch. 12, p. 178*
  Benzene   *Appendix, p. 234*

been linked to development of *acute myelogenous leukemia*. It is probable that a metabolite of benzene, perhaps benzoquinone, is responsible for these effects. Toxicants which damage dividing cells (such as *radiation* or some *anticancer drugs*) also produce bone marrow toxicity.

Rather than producing broad effects on bone marrow, some toxicants may affect one or more blood cells specifically. Several drugs produce decreases in platelet numbers, while others inhibit production of various classes of white blood cells.

Red blood cell levels are affected not only by the actions of toxicants on bone marrow, but also by the action of toxicants on circulating cells. A decrease in the numbers of red blood cells resulting from the destruction of circulating cells is called *hemolytic anemia*. In one type of hemolytic anemia, oxidants such as *phenylhydrazine* or *aniline* produce reactive peroxides which are detoxified through reactions involving the oxidation of glutathione. The oxidized glutathione is then reduced by an enzyme, glutathione reductase, a step which requires NADPH (which is generated in the red blood cell during glycolysis in a series of steps called the hexosemonophosphate shunt). If activity of the oxidants outstrips the ability of the red cell to produce NADPH, then glutathione cannot be reduced, peroxides may accumulate, and oxidative damage to hemoglobin may occur. The decreased solubility of the damaged hemoglobin causes it to precipitate and form visible deposits called *Heinz bodies*. Heinz bodies distort the shape of the red blood cell, often leading to its destruction through hemolysis. Some individuals suffer a genetic deficiency in an enzyme, *glucose-6-phosphate dehydrogenase (G6PD)* which is necessary for NADPH generation. These individuals would be even more susceptible to hemolysis by oxidants than unaffected individuals would be.

Other toxicants, such as the heavy metals *lead* and *mercury*, can cause red blood cell hemolysis through other mechanisms. Lead, for example, increases hemolysis probably through damage to the cell membrane. Lead also affects hemoglobin synthesis, inhibiting the enzyme ALA-D and other enzymes important to heme production. Genetic variations of the enzyme ALA-D between individuals may lead to differences in individual susceptibility to lead.

Effects on Hemoglobin

Some toxicants produce their effects by interfering with the binding of oxygen molecules to hemoglobin. *Carbon monoxide*, for example, binds at the same site on the hemoglobin molecule as does oxygen, and with an affinity 245 times higher. Thus, low levels of carbon monoxide are able to produce significant binding to hemoglobin and resulting displacement of oxygen. Exposure to an atmosphere containing 0.1% carbon monoxide can lead to symptoms such as headache, nausea, tachycardia, and even death from oxygen deprivation in a matter of hours. Opportunities for exposure to carbon monoxide are common, because it is produced during the process of combustion of fossil fuels. Smokers, in fact, may have up to 10% of their hemoglobin saturated with carbon monoxide (as compared to less than 1% in nonsmokers).

Another category of toxicants that can interact with hemoglobin are the *nitrites, nitrates, aromatic amines,* and other nitrogen-containing compounds.

These compounds (or in many cases, their metabolites) can oxidize the heme molecules, converting the iron atom from a ferrous to a ferric state. Ferric iron cannot combine with oxygen, and thus the hemoglobin molecule (now called *methemoglobin*) cannot function normally. Red blood cells have an

NITRATES, NITRITES
see also:
Cellular sites	*Ch. 4, p. 50*
Cardiovascular	
toxicology	*Ch. 8, p. 111*
Water pollution	*Ch. 15, p. 221*
Nitrates	*Appendix, p. 240*

enzyme, methemoglobin reductase, which is capable of reducing methemoglobin. The enzyme does, however, require NADH (which is supplied by glycolysis). A second system for reducing methemoglobin also exists, and can be activated by administration of the compound methylene blue (a dye). This second system requires NADPH (supplied by the pentose phosphate shunt) (Figure 6).

Due to the presence of methemoglobin reductase, methemoglobinemia is not a common problem. One exception is in infants, who have lower levels of methemoglobin reductase than adults, and who may be exposed to nitrates in drinking water (particularly in rural areas).

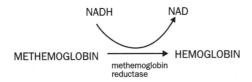

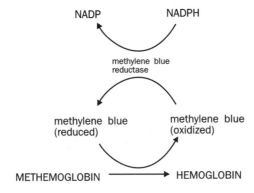

Figure 6   Reduction systems for methemoglobin.

REFERENCES

Fenoglio, J. J., Jr. and Wagner, B. M., Endomyocardial biopsy approach to drug-related heart disease, in *Principles and Methods of Toxicology*, Hayes, A. W., Ed., Raven Press, New York, 1989, chap. 22.

Hanig, J. P. and Herman, E. H., Toxic responses of the heart and vascular systems, in *Casarett and Doull's Toxicology*, Amdur, M. O., Doull, J., and Klaassen, C. D., Eds., Pergamon Press, New York, 1991, chap. 14.

James, R. C., Hematotoxicity: toxic effects in the blood, in *Industrial Toxicology*, Williams, P. L. and Burson, J. L., Eds., Van Nostrand Reinhold, New York, 1985, chap. 4.

Jandl, J. H., Hematologic disorders, in *Occupational Health*, Levy, B. S. and Wegman, D. H., Eds., Little, Brown, and Company, Boston, 1983, chap. 24.

Rosenman, K. D., Cardiovascular disorders, in *Occupational Health*, Levy, B. S. and Wegman, D. H., Eds., Little, Brown, and Company, Boston, 1983, chap. 22.

Smith, R. P., Toxic responses of the blood, in *Casarett and Doull's Toxicology*, Amdur, M. O., Doull, J., and Klaassen, C. D., Eds., Pergamon Press, New York, 1991, chap. 8.

Van Stee, E. W., Cardiovascular toxicology: foundations and scope, in *Cardiovascular Toxicology*, VanStee, E. W., Ed., Raven Press, New York, 1982.

9   NEUROTOXICOLOGY

FUNCTION OF THE NERVOUS SYSTEM

In general, the nervous system has three functions. First of all, specialized cells detect *sensory* information from the environment and then relay that information to other parts of the nervous system. Then another segment of the system directs the *motor* functions of the body, often in direct response to sensory input. Finally, part of the nervous system is involved in processing of information. These *integrative* functions include such things as thought processes, learning, and memory. All of these functions are potentially vulnerable to the actions of toxicants.

ANATOMY AND PHYSIOLOGY OF THE NERVOUS SYSTEM

The nervous system consists of two fundamental anatomical divisions: the *central nervous system* (CNS) and the *peripheral nervous system* (PNS). The CNS includes the brain and spinal cord, while the PNS consists of all other nervous tissue which lies outside the CNS.

The CNS is structurally quite complex, but can be divided into four major areas based on the process of neural development. Within the brain, there is a *forebrain* region which consists of the *cerebrum* (cerebral cortex and basal ganglia), the *thalamus* and the *hypothalamus*. There is also a small *midbrain* region, and a *hindbrain* consisting of the *medulla, pons,* and *cerebellum.* The fourth major area is the *spinal cord* (Figure 1).

The PNS includes both *afferent* nerves which relay sensory information from specialized receptors to the CNS, and *efferent* nerves which relay motor information from the CNS to various muscles and glands. Efferent nerves which carry motor information to skeletal muscles makeup the *somatic* or *voluntary* nervous system, while efferent nerves which carry motor information to smooth muscles, cardiac muscle, and various glands are part of the *autonomic* or *involuntary* nervous system.

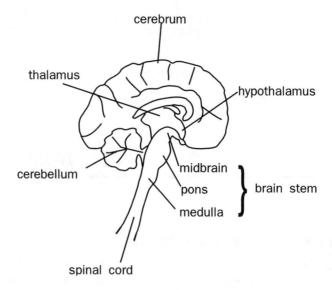

Figure 1   Parts of the central nervous system.

There are two types of cells found within the nervous system: *neurons* and *glial cells*. Neurons are the cells directly responsible for transmission of information. An individual neuron consists of a cell *body* (also called a soma, or perikaryon), and processes called *dendrites* and *axons* (Figure 2). Each part of the neuron has a specific function. The cell body contains a nucleus, mitochondria,

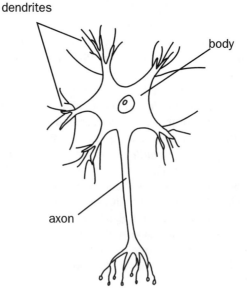

Figure 2
The neuron.

endoplasmic reticulum, and other organelles and is where most cellular metabolism occurs (including virtually all of the protein synthesis). Dendrites are branching extensions of the cell body, specialized for reception of incoming information. Axons transmit information to other neurons. A cell may have many dendrites, but generally has only one axon. Many neurons together form a *nerve*.

Glial cells function as supporting cells. *Astrocytes* provide structural support, and *microglia* are phagocytic (engulfing and digesting dead material and debris, thus removing it from the CNS). *Ependymal* cells line the ventricles (fluid-filled cavities) of the brain. The remaining two types of glial cells are involved in the formation of *myelin*, a lipid-rich substance which covers many axons and aids in efficient conduction of information. These are the *oligodendroglial* cells (which produce myelin in the CNS), and the *Schwann cells* (which produce myelin in the PNS).

Within the nervous system, information is passed along the nets of interconnected neurons by chemical and electrical signals. Within each neuron, the signal is electrical in nature, with each electrical impulse being initiated at the dendrites then traveling through the cell body and down the axon. Communication between neurons, on the other hand, is primarily chemical in nature. Neurons do not physically contact each other—there is a small gap between the axon of one neuron and the dendrite of another. This junction, consisting of the axon, dendrite, and gap between them is called a *synapse*. When an electrical impulse reaches an axon it triggers the release of small molecules called *neurotransmitters* which then migrate across a synaptic gap and bind to protein receptors on the dendrites of the next neuron. This chemical binding, and the conformational change it induces in the receptor, then triggers the start of an electrical impulse in that neuron. In this manner, then, information is relayed throughout the nervous system. Some motor neurons pass their impulse along not to other neurons but to voluntary muscles. This nerve–muscle connection is known as the *neuromuscular junction*.

EFFECTS OF TOXICANTS ON THE NERVOUS SYSTEM— GENERAL PRINCIPLES

The nervous system is a vulnerable target for toxicants due to critical voltages which must be maintained in cells and the all or none responses when voltages reach threshold levels. In addition, the role of the nervous system in directing many critical physiological operations means that any damage may well have significant functional consequences.

The central nervous system does, however, have one major source of protection against injury by toxic chemicals—the blood-brain barrier. Anatomically, the blood-brain barrier consists of modifications to the cells which line capillaries in the brain (*endothelial* cells). These changes (tighter junctions between cells, for example) distinguish CNS endothelial cells from endothelial cells found in other parts of the body. Some glial cells may be a part of the blood-brain barrier, also,

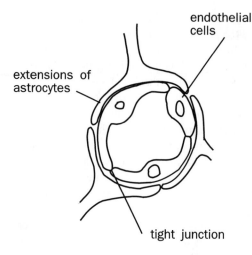

Figure 3
The blood-brain barrier. A combination of tight junctions between endothelial cells and the surrounding of capillaries by extensions of astrocytes prevent easy passage of many molecules from blood into brain tissue.

since long processes from astrocytes are found wrapped around capillaries in many parts of the brain. The functional result of the blood-brain barrier is to keep many blood-borne molecules from entering the central nervous system. Therefore, most toxicants which affect the central nervous system tend to be small, highly lipid soluble, nonpolar molecules—if they were not, they could not diffuse through the barrier.

There are, however, other ways to pass the blood-brain barrier than diffusion. Several specific transport systems are associated with the blood-brain barrier and allow the transport of essential nutrients (such as glucose and amino acids) and ions into the brain, as well as the transport of other molecules out of the brain back into the blood.

Some evidence points to the existence of a metabolic blood-brain barrier as well as an anatomical one. Although tissues of the CNS are low in levels of detoxifying enzymes such as the cytochrome P450 system, there are other enzymes, such as monoamine oxidase or catechol-*O*-methyl transferases that can metabolically change molecules as soon as they cross the endothelium, thus modifying their potential toxic effects.

There are a few areas in the CNS such as the pituitary and the hypothalamus in which the blood-brain barrier is reduced or lacking. Also, some toxicants such as *lead* may damage the barrier. While most of the central nervous system is afforded the protection of the blood-brain barrier, most of the peripheral nervous system is not. This may help explain the different action of toxicants on the two parts of the system. The blood-brain barrier may not only provide a barrier to toxicants, though, but also to therapeutic compounds. For example, an antidote for organophosphate poisoning, 2-PAM, is effective in the peripheral but not the central nervous system, due to its inability to cross the blood-brain barrier. The blood-brain barrier, however, is not well developed at birth, and thus provides less protection in younger organisms.

The effects which toxicants have on the nervous system can be grouped into several categories. These categories will be introduced here, and then explored in more detail in later sections. Some toxicants affect the *passage of electrical impulses* down the axon. These toxicants interfere with the passage of sensory, motor, and also integrative impulses, leading to effects such as paresthesias (abnormal sensations such as tingling or hot or cold sensations), numbness, weakness, and paralysis. Some toxicants *affect synaptic transmission* between neurons, leading to either under- or overstimulation of a part of the nervous system. Toxicants which affect *myelin* also disrupt conduction of the electrical impulse, as do toxicants which *damage neuronal axons*. Exposure to some toxicants can lead to *neuronal cell death* (producing a variety of physiological effects), and the effects of other toxicants are produced through *unknown mechanisms*.

EFFECTS OF TOXICANTS ON ELECTRICAL CONDUCTION

In order to carry out its functions, the nervous system needs to be able to efficiently conduct information from one part of the body to another. As discussed briefly in the introductory chapters, information is passed along from one neuron to another in the form of electrical and chemical impulses. We will now look at this process in more detail and describe how it can be affected by various toxicants.

At rest, a neuron has a *membrane potential* of approximately -70 mV, indicating that there are more negatively charged ions inside the cell (in the intracellular fluid) than there are outside it (in the extracellular fluid). This uneven distribution of charge is caused in part by the fact that, although the membrane is quite permeable to some ions, it is not permeable to many of the large, negatively charged proteins found within the neuron. Thus, these molecules are trapped inside the neuron, contributing to the excess negative charge within.

The membrane potential is also due to the uneven distribution of various ions across the neuronal membrane. This membrane contains several protein channels which allow passage of various ions through the mem-

ION CHANNELS
see also:
    Cellular sites of action   Ch. 4, p. 48

brane. There are channels specific for sodium ions, and channels for potassium ions, among others. The opening of these ion channels depolarizes the membrane potential; changes in the membrane potential also affect the opening and closing of the channels (probably by changing the shape and arrangement of the molecules which form the channel). Because of their reaction to changes in membrane potential, these channels are often called *voltage-gated channels*.

Another component found in the neuronal membrane is an active transport system called the *sodium-potassium pump*. This energy-dependent system simultaneously transports 3 molecules of sodium (a positively charged ion) out of the

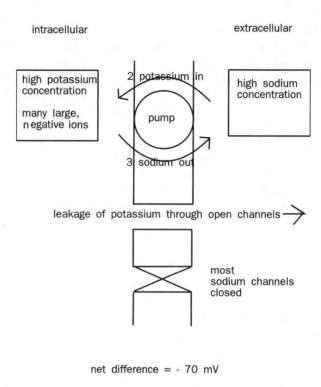

intracellular   extracellular

Figure 4   Resting membrane potential. Differential permeability of the neuronal membrane and the Na⁺/K⁺ pump create a potential difference or voltage across the membrane.

cell and 2 molecules of potassium (also positively charged) into the cell. Some of the potassium which is pumped into the cell will leak back out, because the potassium channels in a resting neuron are usually at least partially open. However, the action of the pump plus the attractive force of the negatively charged molecules trapped within the cell still manage to maintain a higher concentration of potassium inside the cell than outside. The sodium ion channels, unlike the potassium ion channels, are nearly all closed in the resting neuron. Because of this, almost all of the sodium which was pumped out of the cell remains outside the cell.

Chloride ions are also unevenly distributed across the neuronal membrane. Chloride is found in much higher concentrations outside than inside the neuron, probably because of a combination of factors. The negatively charged chloride ion is repulsed by the negatively charged ions within the cell, and may be actively transported outward by a chloride pump, as well. The uneven distribution of chloride, as well as that of sodium and potassium, also contributes to the formation of the negative membrane potential.

The membrane potential of a neuron changes during the propagation of an electrical impulse, or *action potential*. When a neurotransmitter binds to a receptor on a dendrite, it opens sodium channels, making the membrane potential in

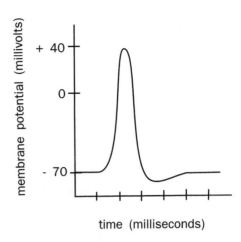

Figure 5
The action potential.

time (milliseconds)

that region less negative (more details on how this happens later on). This change in membrane potential then causes the opening of even more sodium channels (which are, as you remember, voltage gated) in a chain reaction. The action potential occurs when this reaction builds to the point that it becomes self-sustaining. At that point, the *threshold*, the membrane potential rapidly changes from –70 mV to +30 mV (a process called *depolarization*). This change in potential then spreads rapidly across the entire neuronal membrane. Almost as soon as a part of the membrane is depolarized, though, *repolarization* begins. Sodium channels close, and the opening of potassium channels allows positive potassium ions to leave the cell and thus restore the negative membrane potential. The sodium-potassium pump will then restore intra- and extracellular levels of sodium and potassium to their original levels. During the process of repolarization the neuron is said to be in a *refractory* state during which it cannot conduct another action potential.

A number of neurotoxicants can interfere with the propagation of electrical impulses. *Tetrodotoxin* (TTX) is a toxicant of biological origin, found in a number of frogs, fish, and other species including the blue-ringed octopus of Australia, and the puffer fish which is a popular food in Japan. Tetrodotoxin blocks the action

TTX, STX
see also:
Cellular sites of action   *Ch. 4, p. 40*
Cardiovascular
    toxicology   *Ch. 8, p. 106*
TTX, STX   *Appendix, p. 246*

potential by binding to a site on the outside of the neuronal membrane and blocking the sodium channels. Effects of tetrodotoxin include motor weakness and paresthesias. Higher doses may cause paralysis, not only of skeletal (voluntary) muscle, but also of smooth muscle in blood vessels which may then lead to severe hypotension and circulatory failure. Most tetrodotoxin poisonings occur in people who have eaten improperly prepared puffer fish. Although tetrodotoxin concentration in the fish

intracellular   extracellular

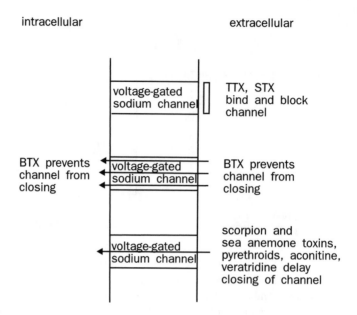

Figure 6   Actions of toxicants on ion channels in the neuronal membrane.

muscle is relatively low, levels may be high (up to 10 mg/g) in other organs such as the liver. The LD_{50} of tetrodotoxin in mice is around 300 μg/kg.

Another biological toxin that blocks sodium channels is saxitoxin (STX). Saxitoxin is produced by organisms called dinoflagellates (of the genus *Gonyaulax* among others). These organisms serve as a food source for various shellfish and fish. Although many fish are killed by exposure to this toxin, many shellfish are not susceptible and may accumulate a milligram or more of the toxin. Then, the shellfish may be eaten by unsuspecting humans who may then become ill or perhaps even die. To prevent this, shellfish harvesting may be prohibited in affected areas during periods of dinoflagellate "blooms" (large increases in population).

A third biological toxin is *batrachotoxin* (BTX), found in South American frogs, and used as an arrow poison. Although batrachotoxin (like tetrodotoxin and saxitoxin) prevents the passage of nerve impulses, its mechanism of action is somewhat different. Batrachotoxin increases the permeability of the resting neuronal membrane to sodium by preventing closing of the sodium channels. Thus, the membrane potential (which depends in part on uneven distribution of sodium across the membrane) cannot properly develop, and the action potential cannot be created or propagate. Batrachotoxin can act from either the inside or outside of the membrane, which is probably more a reflection of its high degree of lipid solubility than an indication of where on the channel it is binding. Batrachotoxin also modifies the selectivity of the channel (its ability to exclude ions other than sodium) It is extremely toxic: less than 200 μg may be fatal to a human.

Several *scorpion and sea anemone toxins* have a similar action to batrachotoxin, delaying the closing of sodium channels. These peptides act from the outside of the membrane, and can prolong action potential duration from several milliseconds to several seconds by binding strongly to open sodium channels.

Pyrethroids (a class of synthetic insecticides), and some *organochlorine* insecticides (including DDT) as well as the plant alkaloids *aconitine* and *veratridine* also delay closing of sodium channels. These compounds probably act at different sites, though, than either batrachotoxin or the scorpion or sea anemone toxins.

PESTICIDES	
see also:	
Water pollution	**Ch. 15, p. 215**
Pyrethroids	**Appendix, p. 246**
Organochlorine	
pesticides	**Appendix, p. 241**

EFFECTS OF TOXICANTS ON SYNAPTIC FUNCTION

There are two types of synapses in the nervous system: the synapse between two nerve cells and the synapse between a nerve and a muscle cell or gland. Both, however, operate on similar principles.

At a synapse where two neurons come together (Figure 7), the axonal membrane is termed the *presynaptic* membrane, the dendritic membrane is termed the *postsynaptic* membrane, and the gap between them the *synaptic gap*. The dendrites and cell body of any one neuron may receive inputs from many axons.

At some synapses, the electrical impulse in the presynaptic neuron is communicated to the postsynaptic membrane directly through electrical current. In most cases, though, communication between the pre- and postsynaptic neurons is chemical in nature. When an electrical impulse reaches the end of the presynaptic axon, the change in membrane potential triggers the release of a chemical messenger called a neurotransmitter. The neurotransmitter then diffuses across the synaptic gap to bind to special *receptor* molecules on the postsynaptic membrane. This binding affects the membrane potential of the postsynaptic neuron. Neurotransmitters and neurohormones affect only neurons containing the corresponding selective receptor protein, thus, they do not excite all neurons.

There are two general types of neuroreceptors: excitatory and inhibitory. Each is activated by specific ligands. Binding of neurotransmitters to *excitatory* neuroreceptors opens ion channels, allowing cations (positive ions such as sodium) to enter the cell, and thus making the membrane potential a little less negative. This change lasts for only a few milliseconds, after which the potential returns to its original level. If enough neurotransmitters are released simultaneously, however, many ion channels will be opened and the effects will add up in a process called *summation*. As more and more sodium channels open, the mem-

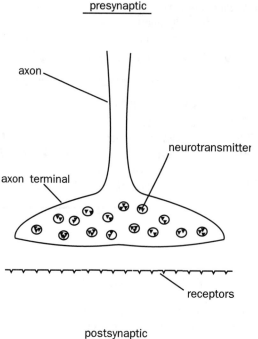

presynaptic

axon

neurotransmitter

axon terminal

receptors

postsynaptic

Figure 7
The cholinergic synapse.

brane potential becomes less and less negative, until finally an action potential may be generated.

Other neurotransmitters bind to *inhibitory* neuroreceptors. Binding of these neurotransmitters to their receptors opens potassium and chloride channels. This allows more potassium to leave the cell and chloride to enter, making the membrane potential even more negative and thus preventing the initiation of an action potential.

There are many different neurotransmitter substances in the nervous system. Generally, each neuron manufactures and *releases* only one single type of neurotransmitter. A single neuron may, however, *receive* inputs from several different types of neurons, each releasing a different neurotransmitter. The results may be both excitatory and inhibitory, depending on the types of specific receptors present in the neuron. The major types of neurotransmitters are *acetylcholine*, the *biogenic amines*, the *amino acids*, and the *neuropeptides*. Lately, evidence has also accumulated that *nitric oxide* a gas, may also be a neurotransmitter.

Acetylcholine

Acetylcholine (ACh) is an important neurotransmitter in the autonomic nervous system (the system which controls involuntary muscle movement). The autonomic nervous system has two branches: the *sympathetic* and the *parasympa-thetic*. The sympathetic and parasympathetic branches control many of the same muscles and glands, but the effects of each branch on those muscles and glands differ greatly. The physiological state of the body reflects the balance between the two influences. Stimulation of the sympathetic branch leads to what is often called the "fight or flight" response: tachycardia (increase in heart rate), dilation of bron-chioles, dilation of the pupil, constriction of peripheral blood vessels, and decrease in digestive activity. Parasympathetic stimulation leads to bradycardia (decrease in heart rate), constriction of bronchioles, constriction of the pupil, increase in peristalsis (activity of digestive smooth muscle), and increase in secretions.

In both branches, the connection between the central nervous system and the muscle or gland which is to be controlled consists of two neurons. The first neu-ron (the *preganglionic*) connects the CNS with a group of nerve cells called a *gan-glion*, the second (*postganglionic*) neuron originates in the ganglion and connects with the muscle or gland it controls. Acetylcholine is released by the pregan-glionic neurons of both branches, and by the postganglionic neurons of the parasympathetic branch. Acetylcholine is also released by the neurons that con-trol voluntary muscle movement, and is released by neurons in areas of the cen-tral nervous system as well (Figure 8).

Acetylcholine is synthesized within the neuron from the molecules acetyl CoA and choline. The rate of synthesis is dependent on the supply of choline, which is taken up from outside the neuron by a sodium-dependent transport mech-anism. A molecule called *hemicholinium*, (HC-3) is able to block this transport process, leading to a reduction in acetylcholine levels. Acetylcholine is stored in the neuron, perhaps in membrane-bound droplets called vesicles or perhaps else-where in the cytoplasm. Release of "packets" of acetylcholine molecules from the axon is a calcium-dependent process which occurs regularly even when the neu-ron is resting. A much larger, synchronized release of the neurotransmitter is trig-gered by the rapid influx of calcium which accompanies action potential-induced changes in the membrane potential.

One of the most deadly toxicants known, *botulinum toxin*, (with an LD_{50} in some animals as low as 10 ng/kg) binds to the nerve axon and interferes with the release of acetylcholine. Botulinum toxin is actually a group of at least seven dif-ferent toxic proteins produced by the bacterium *Clostridium botulinum*, which can grow on improperly processed or mishandled foods. Because this bacterium is anaerobic (doesn't use oxygen), it can grow quite well in sealed containers, and the majority of cases of botulism poisoning in the U.S. are related to consumption of home-canned foods. The symptoms of botulism poisoning reflect the interrup-tion of impulse transmission by neurons which use acetylcholine, and include muscle weakness and paralysis (neuromuscular junction effects), blurred vision (autonomic effects), and other effects such as nausea and diarrhea.

Once released from the axon terminal, acetylcholine molecules migrate across the synaptic gap and bind to the acetylcholine receptors found on the post-synaptic membrane in cholinergic synapses. There are two different types of

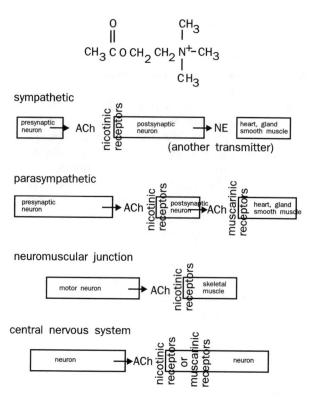

Figure 8   The neurotransmitter acetylcholine and its locations in the nervous system. Types of cholinergic receptors are also shown.

receptors which respond to acetylcholine: *nicotinic* receptors (named on the basis of their response to nicotine) and *muscarinic* receptors (named on the basis of their response to the drug muscarine). Nicotinic receptors are found on neurons in autonomic ganglia of both branches, and on skeletal muscle. Muscarinic receptors are found where neurons of the parasympathetic system connect to smooth muscle and glands (Figure 8). When acetylcholine binds to the nicotinic receptor, it directly opens a cation channel, immediately allowing an influx of cations and making the membrane potential less negative. Action at the muscarinic receptor is somewhat slower. When acetylcholine binds to this receptor, a group of proteins called G proteins are activated, initiating a series of biochemical changes (involving "second messenger" compounds such as cyclic AMP) which then ultimately regulates the opening and closing of calcium and potassium channels.

Compounds such as nicotine and muscarine are cholinergic *agonists*. That means that they bind to the nicotinic or muscarinic receptor and mimic the effects of acetylcholine. Other compounds also bind to the nicotinic or muscarinic receptor, but with different results. Instead of mimicking acetylcholine, they compete with acetylcholine for binding and *block* the receptor, preventing the initiation of

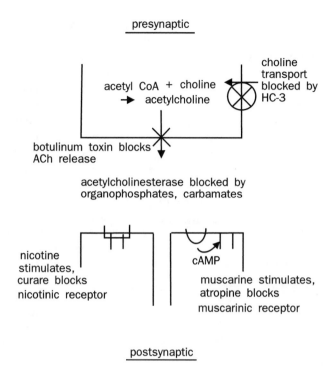

presynaptic

acetyl CoA + choline → acetylcholine

choline transport blocked by HC-3

botulinum toxin blocks ACh release

acetylcholinesterase blocked by organophosphates, carbamates

nicotine stimulates, curare blocks nicotinic receptor

cAMP

muscarine stimulates, atropine blocks muscarinic receptor

postsynaptic

Figure 9 Effects of various toxicants on the cholinergic system.

an action potential in the postsynaptic neuron. One example of such a nicotinic *antagonist* is curare. The term curare actually includes a number of different arrow poisons used by South American Indians. These poisons contain a number of alkaloids such as d-tubocurarine which bind to and block the nicotinic receptor. Effects of blocking the nicotinic receptors at the neuromuscular junction include motor weakness and paralysis. Duration is brief, and reversible, but death may occur from paralysis of the diaphragm muscle (which is essential to breathing). Effects which result from blocking of receptors at the ganglia include decreases in blood pressure and heart rate. Because of their effects, these compounds are used in conjunction with general anesthetics to induce muscle relaxation during surgery.

Atropine, a muscarinic blocker, is found in the plants *Atropa belladonna* ("Deadly nightshade") and *Datura stramonium* ("Jimson weed"). Known since ancient times, *Atropa* is named for Atropos, the Fate who cuts thread of life; belladonna means "beautiful lady," a reflection of the plant's cosmetic use to widen the pupil of the eye. Another muscarinic blocker, *scopolamine*, is found in the plant *Hyoscamus niger* ("Henbane"). Blockade of muscarinic receptors blocks the effect of the parasympathetic neurons on muscles and glands and leads to an autonomic system imbalance in favor of the sympathetic branch. As little as 2.0 mg of atropine in a human can produce tachycardia, dilation of the pupils, dilation of bronchioles, decrease in peristalsis, and decrease in secretions such as saliva. Atropine also has some effects on the central nervous system, producing general excitation with small doses, and depression with larger doses. Both atropine and scopolamine may be hallucinogenic. Much larger doses are necessary to affect the CNS than to produce autonomic effects, probably due to the exclusion of the compounds by the blood-brain barrier.

ACETYLCHOLINESTERASE

see also:

Biotransformation	***Ch. 3, p. 24***
Cellular sites of action	***Ch. 4, p. 39***

After acetylcholine has been released and binding to the receptors has occurred there must be a way to inactivate the neurotransmitter. Otherwise, receptors would continue to be stimulated, and action potentials would continue to be produced long after the original impulse had passed. In the case of acetylcholine, the remaining molecules are hydrolyzed in a reaction catalyzed by an enzyme called acetylcholinesterase (AChase). Hydrolysis of acetylcholine occurs in three steps: reversible binding to the enzyme, acetylation of a serine residue at the enzyme active site (yielding choline), and deacetylation on attack by a hydroxyl ion (yielding acetate). *Organophosphates* (OPs) and *carbamates* are two

ORGANOPHOSPHATES

see also:

Cellular sites of action	***Ch. 4, p. 39***
Neurotoxicology	***Ch. 9, p. 130, 137***
Water pollution	***Ch. 15, p. 217***
Organophosphates	***Appendix, p. 242***

classes of pesticides that can bind to and inhibit acetylcholinesterase. Because inhibition is reversible in the case of carbamates, their action is of short duration. Inhibition by OPs, however, is a different matter. The bond formed between the acetylcholinesterase and most OPs is quite stable, and only slowly reversible. In fact, recovery from poisoning by some OPs (such as military nerve agents) may depend on synthesis of new acetylcholinesterase.

Effects of OP and carbamate poisoning reflect overstimulation of the parasympathetic nervous system and include slowing of heart rate, constriction of the pupils, bronchoconstriction, and increase in secretions (four classic symptoms are salivation, lacrimation, urination, and defecation). Overstimulation at the neuromuscular junction produces twitching and cramps; central effects include anxiety, restlessness, and confusion which can lead to coma. Death is usually by respiratory failure brought on by paralysis of respiratory muscles and inhibition of the central nervous system centers which control respiration.

The oral LD_{50} for organophosphates range from one to several thousand mg/kg. Antidotal treatment is with atropine, which blocks muscarinic receptors. In addition, a molecule called *pralidoxime* (also called 2-PAM) helps accelerate the reversal of acetylcholinesterase inhibition.

Biogenic Amines

A second group of neurotransmitters and neurohormones is the biogenic amines, which includes the neurotransmitters norepinephrine, epinephrine, dopamine, serotonin, and histamine. *Norepinephrine* is the neurotransmitter released by the postganglionic neurons of the sympathetic nervous system. It is also released by some neurons of the central nervous system. Many of these norepinephrine-releasing neurons (as well as many neurons which release *epinephrine*, many that release *dopamine*, and many that release *serotonin*) originate in the medulla, pons, or midbrain (a grouping of areas which is commonly called the *brain stem*) and lead to many other areas of the brain. *Histamine*-releasing neurons are found in highest concentrations in the hypothalamus.

Norepinephrine, epinephrine, and dopamine together are known as the *catecholamines*. Toxicants can interfere with this group of neurotransmitters through many of the mechanisms we have already discussed. The drug *reserpine*, for example, interferes with the storage of biogenic amines in the axon, leading to a shortage of these neurotransmitters. This results in a decrease in sympathetic

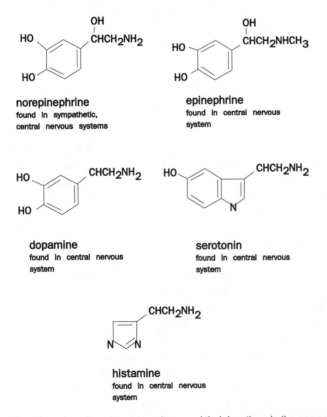

Figure 10 The biogenic amine neurotransmitters and their locations in the nervous system.

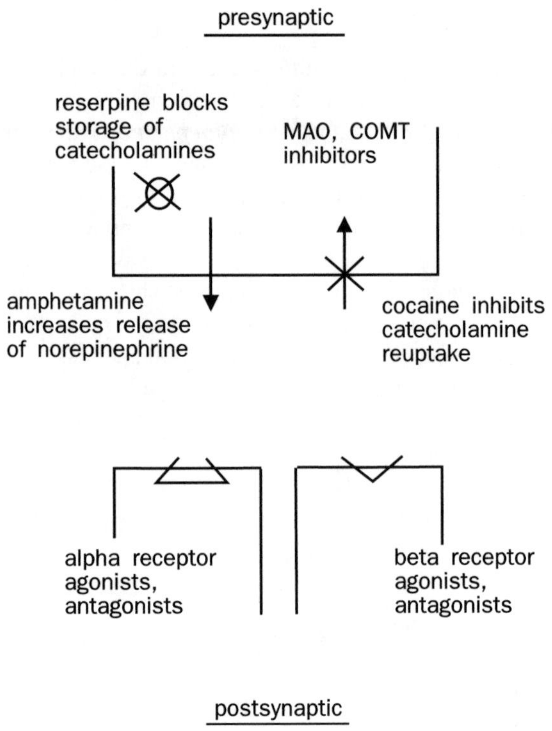

presynaptic

Figure 11 Effects of various toxicants on the biogenic amines.

activity (producing slowing of heart rate), an increase in digestive activity, and an increase in secretions. *Amphetamine*, on the other hand, exerts part of its stimulatory effects through promoting increased release of norepinephrine.

As is the case with acetylcholine, there are two major categories of receptors which respond to the catecholamines: *alpha* and *beta* adrenergic receptors. They can be differentiated on the basis of their relative sensitivities to norepinephrine and epinephrine. Alpha and beta receptors can be further subdivided into alpha one and alpha two, beta one and beta two populations. Alpha one receptors are found on smooth muscles and glands while alpha two receptors are thought to be involved in feedback inhibition of various neurons throughout the nervous system. Beta one receptors are found in heart tissue; beta two receptors (like alpha one receptors) are found on smooth muscle and glands.

Many compounds interact with catecholamine receptors, some as agonists (stimulating the sympathetic nervous system) and some as antagonists (depressing the sympathetic nervous system). Many nasal decongestants are alpha agonists which work by constricting blood vessels of the nose. Alpha agonists can also be used to treat hypotension (low blood pressure) such as accompanies shock. Many beta two agonists are extremely useful in widening of bronchial airways constricted by asthma; because these compounds are specific for beta two and do not stimulate beta one receptors there are no side effects such as increased heart rate. *Amphetamine* stimulates both alpha and beta receptors and of course is a CNS stimulant as well.

Several drugs act as alpha blockers, producing decreases in blood pressure, increases in activity of gastrointestinal muscles, and nasal stuffiness due to dilation of blood vessels. One group of compounds that interacts with alpha receptors in a complex manner are the *ergot alkaloids*. These compounds are produced by the fungus *Claviceps purpurea*, which grows on rye and other grains. Its effects have been known for centuries (epidemics of ergot poisoning were fairly common during the Middle Ages). Some ergot alkaloids act as partial agonists and others as antagonists of alpha receptors. Ergot alkaloids stimulate smooth muscle contraction, and one of the predominant symptoms of ergotism was gangrene of the extremities (caused by constriction of the smooth muscle of blood vessels in the arms and legs). Spontaneous abortion due to stimulation of uterine muscle was also common. These drugs are still used in treatment of migraine (which may result in part from increases in blood flow in cranial arteries).

Beta receptor blocking drugs such as *propranolol* are widely used to manage cardiovascular disorders due to their ability to decrease both heart rate and blood pressure. Other drugs have been developed recently which are more specific for beta one receptors, thus eliminating the side effect of bronchoconstriction which would occur if beta two receptors are also blocked.

Deactivation of the catecholamines following their release from the axon is achieved through a different mechanism than inactivation of acetylcholine. Instead of being enzymatically broken down, catecholamines are returned to the axon through a *reuptake mechanism*. Catecholamine reuptake requires sodium and potassium and is energy dependent. Inhibition of reuptake (by *cocaine*, for example) may lead to overstimulation of the postsynaptic neuron. Within the axon, catecholamines can be broken down by two enzymes: *monoamine oxidase (MAO)* and *catechol-O-methyltransferase (COMT)*. Inhibitors of these enzymes (for example the antidepressant drug chlorpromazine) can increase levels of catecholamines in brain.

As for effects of toxicants on the remaining biogenic amines, histamine and serotonin, little is known. There are specific receptors for both serotonin and histamine in the brain, and there is conflicting evidence as to whether some hallucinogenic drugs such as *LSD* may interact with serotonin receptors. Like the catecholamines, serotonin is inactivated by reuptake, but through a separate reuptake mechanism. No reuptake process for histamine has been found.

Amino Acid Neurotransmitters

Probably the most significant amino acid neurotransmitter is *gamma-aminobutyric acid (GABA)*. GABA is an inhibitory transmitter, produced by neurons throughout the nervous system and acting only at the inhibitory GABA receptor and chloride ion channel. It is found in particularly high concentrations within the cerebellum and spinal cord, and in cells originating in the hippocampus and leading to the midbrain. Like most neurotransmitters, GABA is manufactured and stored in the presynaptic neuron and following release binds to a postsynaptic receptor. GABA binding triggers an increase in chloride permeability, allowing chloride to enter the neuron and making the membrane potential more negative. Reuptake of GABA occurs both in the presynaptic neuron and nearby glial cells.

GABAergic pathways seem to be important in control of emotions. The *benzodiazepines* (antianxiety drugs better known by trade names such as Valium and Librium) interact with GABA through a mechanism that is not yet clear. Although they seem to mimic the effects of GABA, they are ineffective if GABA itself is not present. *Picrotoxin*, a powerful stimulant derived from the seeds of an East Indian plant, antagonizes the effects of GABA and also blocks the action of benzodiazepines. The inhibitory effects of GABA may also be important in motor control. Loss of GABAergic neurons occurs in the genetic disorder *Huntington's Disease*, and may be responsible for the involuntary movements (chorea) characteristic of the disease. The cyclodiene insecticides dieldrin and chlordane block the GABA receptor.

Another inhibitory transmitter is the amino acid glycine. Glycine acts primarily in the brain stem and spinal cord. *Tetanus toxin* binds to presynaptic membranes and prevents release of glycine, while *strychnine* (lethal dose in humans of 1 mg/kg), a powerful convulsant, binds to and blocks the postsynaptic glycine receptor. Antagonism of glycine's inhibitory effect leads to the sustained muscle contraction characteristic of both toxicants.

Glutamate and *aspartate* are excitatory amino acids. *Kainic acid* is a glutamate agonist which kills neurons, as can glutamate itself in large concentrations. Mechanisms of neuronal death due to "excitotoxic" effects of glutamine and related amino acids will be discussed later in this chapter.

Neuroactive Peptides

The neuropeptides differ from the other transmitters in the nervous system. Neuropeptides act at much lower concentrations, and their actions last longer. In addition, neuropeptides are generally made in the neuronal cell body rather than in the axon. Like other neurotransmitters, neuropeptides may affect membrane potential, or they may be released along with a neurotransmitter and alter its release or binding.

There are probably 50 to 100 neuropeptides (Table 1); one of the better known groups is the *opioid peptides*. This category includes the *enkephalins* and *endorphins*. Several different opioid receptors occur throughout the central nervous system, and may have inhibitory effects on pathways involved in the transmission of pain impulses. In at least one type of receptor, binding of the peptide to the receptor is linked to the opening of potassium channels through the media-

TABLE 1   Some Types of Neuroactive Peptides, Categorized by
Localization in the Body

Gastrointestinal-related peptides (most found both in the brain and neurons innervating the gastrointestinal tract)	VIP, CCK, substance P, enkephalins, gastrin, neurotensin, insulin, glucagon, bombesin
Hypothalamic-releasing hormones	TRH, LHRH, GH, GHRH, somatostatin
Pituitary peptides	ACTH, endorphin, alpha-MSH, prolactin, LH, GH, thyrotropin
Others	Anglotensin II, bradykinin, oxytocin, vasopressin

tion of a 2nd messenger, cAMP. Other receptors may act presynaptically, controlling calcium channels to decrease release of a neurotransmitter.

The opioid peptides are named for *opium*, a drug derived from the juice of the opium poppy. Opium itself consists of many different compounds including *morphine* and *codeine*, both of which, although they are not peptides, interact with opioid receptors. *Heroin* is a chemical derivative of morphine. Although a few milligrams of morphine or related opioid agonists produce the clinically useful effects of drowsiness and pain relief, they also produce euphoria and have an equally significant history of recreational usage. *Tolerance* to these drugs develops with continued usage: in other words, progressively higher doses are necessary to produce the same physiological effects. *Naloxone* is an opioid receptor antagonist which can block effects of both endogenous peptides and opioid drugs.

AXONOPATHIES

Another potentially vulnerable part of the neuron is the *axon*. The axon projects from the cell body and has a *proximal* section (nearest the cell body) and a *distal* section (containing the end of the axon, or *axon terminal*). These terms are relative: there is no distinct point of division between the two regions.

Unlike the cell body, the axon has limited metabolic capabilities. Most of the molecules that are needed in the axon must be made in the cell body. These molecules are then transported down the axon, often traveling considerable distances (several feet for some motor neurons of the spinal cord). Transport originating in the cell body and moving down the axon is called *anterograde* transport. Other materials may be returned to the cell body from the axon, in a movement called *retrograde* transport.

There are two types of systems involved in axonal transport. The first system is called *slow transport* or *"axoplasmic flow."* Slow transport moves at the rate of 1 mm/day and is strictly anterograde in direction, with no retrograde motion. Most axonal proteins are moved by slow transport, including many enzymes as well as structural proteins such as *microtubules, microfilaments*, and *neurofilaments*. The mechanism of slow transport is unknown: new material seems to displace that

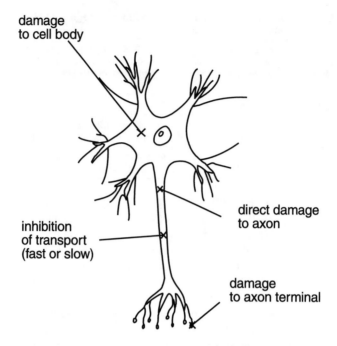

Figure 12   Potential targets for production of axonopathies.

material in front in a process which has been compared to toothpaste moving through the tube.

The second type of transport is *fast* or *axonal transport*. Fast transport moves substances at the much more rapid rate of about 400 mm/day, and can be either anterograde or retrograde in direction. Fast transport distributes membrane components from the cell body to the axon and also returns used membrane components to the cell body for recycling. Fast transport can also move substances absorbed at the axon terminal up to the cell body. Some viruses, including herpes viruses and toxins such as tetanus toxin are thought to enter the cell body in this manner.

The mechanism of fast transport probably involves some or all of the structural elements of the neuron: the microtubules, microfilaments, and neurofilaments. According to one current theory, microtubules form a "track" along the axon. Materials to be moved are attached to and pulled along the track by molecules called kinesins. Studies of the mechanisms of both slow and fast transport are often carried out by radiolabeling molecules and monitoring their progress down the axon.

Axonopathies, damage to the axon, are most common in the peripheral nervous system, and the resulting sensory and motor dysfunction is often referred to as a *neuropathy*. Axonopathies are generally categorized as either proximal or distal. Proximal axonopathies are characterized by a swelling of the proximal axon (called a *giant axonal swelling*). A synthetic aminonitrile compound, *IDPN*, is the only known chemical which produces a proximal axonopathy. IDPN blocks slow transport, but in spite of this, the cell body continues to make proteins. This leads to an accumulation of neurofilaments, and results in the giant axonal swelling. The distal portions of the axon, deprived of necessary structural proteins, then degenerate. Breakdown of myelin (which will be discussed later in this chapter) may also occur around the swelling, probably as a result of the axonal disruption. Giant axonal swellings are associated with the neurological disease *amyotrophic lateral sclerosis (ALS)*. The cause of this disease is uncertain, but some evidence has indicated that environmental factors may be involved.

Distal axonopathies involve pathological changes in the distal portions of axons. This damage varies with the toxicant producing the change, but may include swelling, damage to mitochondria, and accumulation of neurofilaments. Like proximal axonopathies, distal axonopathies are also often accompanied by disintegration of myelin. Because damage often appears in the axon terminal first, these axonopathies are also sometimes called "dying-back neuropathies." Distal axonopathies may follow a single exposure to some toxicants, or may be a result of chronic exposure. Even following a single acute exposure, though, the actual onset of symptoms is unlikely to occur prior to a week following the exposure.

There are several hypotheses concerning the cause of distal axonopathies. One possibility is damage to the cell body of the neuron. If synthesis of cell products such as structural proteins is affected, any shortfall in availability of these products is likely to be found first in the more distal portions of the axon (the end of the line for axonal transport). However, cell body damage has been observed in only a few studies, and may well be the result and not the cause of the axonopathy. In addition, peripheral neurons may regenerate following axonopathy, an event which would be unlikely if the neuronal cell body itself was damaged. An alternative hypothesis is that the axonopathy is due to damage to the axon itself, perhaps initiating at the axon terminal. Finally, effects on transport mechanism(s) may be the cause. It is probable that there is no one single cause, but that different toxicants may act through different mechanisms.

Among the toxicants that produce distal axonopathies are a group of compounds already discussed, the *organophosphates*. In the early 1920s and 1930s neuropathies were reported in tuberculosis patients treated with the organophosphate compound phosphocreosote. Also during that period, cases of "Ginger

---

ORGANOPHOSPHATES
see also:
Cellular sites of action	*Ch. 4, p. 39*
Neurotoxicology	*Ch. 9, p. 130*
Water pollution	*Ch. 15, p. 217*
Organophosphates	*Appendix, p. 242*

Jake" paralysis were traced to ingestion of ginger extract still containing traces of the organophosphates used to make the extract. The neuropathy may occur following either acute exposure to high levels or chronic exposure to lower levels.

Symptoms begin 1 to 2 weeks after acute exposure, and typically include weakness and perhaps even paralysis of the lower limbs. Recovery is slow and seldom complete. Not all species are sensitive to organophosphate-induced neuropathies; those that are sensitive include humans, cats, sheep, and many birds (much experimental work is done using chickens as models).

The mechanism of action of organophosphate axonopathy is not entirely clear. Since the axonopathy is produced by some (but not all) of the acetylcholinesterase-inhibiting organophosphates, some researchers believe that inhibition of a related enzyme (a different esterase) may be involved. Many organophosphates which produce the delayed neuropathy do bind to a molecule with esteratic activity. This molecule has been called "neurotoxic esterase," and although binding to this molecule appears in many cases to be correlated with toxicity, the function of the esterase itself and potential consequences of its inhibition remain unclear.

Some compounds which produce distal axonopathies appear to act primarily by inhibiting axonal transport. One example is *acrylamide*, which blocks slow and possibly fast transport. Another is the compound *2,5-hexanedione* (a metabolite of the solvents *n*-hexane and methyl *n*-butyl ketone). Chronic exposure to these solvents, used in glues and cleaning fluids, leads to accumulation of neurofilaments in the distal portions of the axon, followed by disruption of myelin. The resulting sensory disturbances and motor weakness is sometimes called "gluesniffer's neuropathy." Recovery is generally complete in mild cases, but some impairment may remain in severe cases (perhaps due to involvement of central nervous system neurons).

Chronic exposure to the solvents *carbon disulfide* or *ethanol* can also lead to distal axonopathy.

MYELINOPATHIES

The axons of some neurons in both the central and peripheral nervous systems are covered by an insulating substance called *myelin*. In the central nervous system, myelin is formed when an *oligodendroglial* cell sends out a process which wraps tightly around a segment of the neuronal axon (Figure 13). The myelin-forming cells in the peripheral nervous system are called *Schwann cells*. Unlike oligodendroglial cells which can only wrap one axon, one Schwann cell may send out several processes and contribute segments of myelin to many different axons. In both the central and peripheral nervous systems there are gaps between myelinated segments of an axon. These gaps are called *nodes of Ranvier*. Electrical conduction in myelinated axons is fundamentally the same as in unmyelinated, except that changes in membrane potential occur only at the nodes. Thus the impulse "jumps" from one node to the next in a process called *saltatory conduction* (Figure 14). Saltatory conduction is both faster and more efficient than the continuous conduction which occurs in unmyelinated neurons.

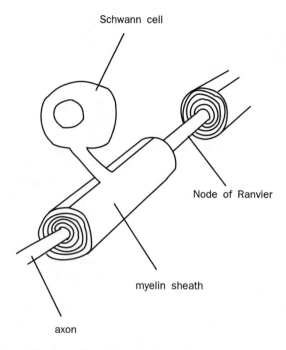

Figure 13 A myelinated axon in the peripheral nervous system.

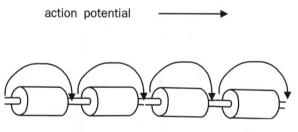

Figure 14 Saltatory conduction in a myelinated axon.

Not surprisingly, the composition of the myelin sheath is similar to that of a typical cell membrane. Myelin contains some water and protein, but consists mostly of lipids (cholesterol, phospholipids, galactosphingolipid).

Damage to myelin interferes with normal function of the nervous system in much the same ways as damage to axons or interference with electrical conduction. Damage to myelin may block conduction completely, or may delay or reduce the amplitude of action potentials (perhaps through transition from saltatory to continuous conduction or through increase in the length of the refractory period). Symptoms of this include numbness, weakness, and paralysis. In addition, action potentials may arise spontaneously in demyelinated neurons, causing paresthesias. Remyelination of demyelinated axons can and does occur.

Some toxicants appear to produce myelinopathy through direct effects on myelin rather than damage to axons or oligodendroglial and Schwann cells. More than 1000 people were exposed to one such compound, *triethyltin*, in France in 1954, through contamination of a supposed antibacterial preparation. Triethyltin is highly lipid soluble, and also binds directly to sites within the myelin. Dosages as low as 6 mg/kg lead to splitting of the myelin sheath and production of large fluid-filled vacuoles within the myelin. This accumulation of fluids is called *edema*.

Another highly lipid soluble compound with strikingly similar effects to triethyltin is *hexachlorophene* (HCP). Hexachlorophene is an excellent antibacterial agent, and was at one time widely used. Studies on premature infants washed with hexachlorophene, however, showed that some had suffered damage to myelin in both the central and peripheral nervous system. Effects of hexachlorophene are generally reversible, as are effects of triethyltin.

LEAD
see also:
Reproductive toxicology ***Ch. 6, p. 75***
Cardiovascular toxicology ***Ch. 8, p. 114***
Neurotoxicology ***Ch. 9, p. 143***
Immunology ***Ch. 12, p. 180***
Water pollution ***Ch. 15, p. 222***
Lead ***Appendix, p. 239***

Although *lead* also causes demyelination, its effects are limited to the peripheral nervous system. In addition, the cause of the demyelination is probably quite different than with hexachlorophene or triethyltin. Swelling and other morphological changes are seen in the Schwann cells along with damage to myelin, indicating that lead is probably damaging the Schwann cell itself.

A human disease of unknown etiology that affects myelin is *multiple sclerosis*. This disease usually strikes young adults between 20 and 40 years of age, with symptoms of sensory disturbances and motor weakness. Pathological changes occur within the central nervous system, and include degeneration of myelin and its replacement by plaques of astrocytes (another type of glial cell). The disease is cyclic, with relapses and improvements probably coinciding with periods of demyelination and remyelination. Some evidence has indicated that there may be a genetic component involved in predisposition toward acquiring the disease; other hypotheses focus on viral involvement or immune system dysfunction. Possibly, all three factors may contribute. For example, a particular viral infection may trigger an immune reaction which destroys not only the invading virus but also attacks some of the proteins found in myelin.

EFFECTS DIRECTLY ON NEURONS

Finally, some neurotoxicants exert their effects directly on the cell bodies of neurons. Neurons which have been damaged by toxicants often show structural changes such as swelling and breakdown of organelles such as rough endoplasmic reticulum and mitochondria or damage to synaptic membranes. Chronic exposure to some neurotoxicants results in accumulations of filaments which are then called *neurofibrillary tangles*. These tangles also result from some diseases such as *Alzheimer's disease*. Functional changes in the damaged neuron can include decreases in protein synthesis and oxidative metabolism. These changes may then affect the ability of the neuron to transmit impulses, and may ultimately lead to cell death.

One cytotoxic neurotoxicant is the excitatory neurotransmitter *glutamate*. Low levels of *monosodium glutamate* (MSG), a popular food additive, produces in some people a group of symptoms often called "Chinese Restaurant Syndrome." These sensitive individuals may react to as little as 1 to 2 g of MSG with burning or tingling sensations in the upper body, and occasionally even chest discomfort. These symptoms are probably produced by interaction of glutamate with the peripheral nervous system. Exposure to high levels of this neurotransmitter produces central nervous system effects such as convulsions or death.

Glutamate seems to attack dendrites and cell bodies of neurons, probably because that is where the glutamate receptors are located. The constant depolarization produced by glutamate probably overstimulates affected neurons, and cell death may result from exhaustion of energy supplies. Research has focused on a class of glutamate receptors called the NMDA receptor (named for the fact that the receptors respond to N-methyl-D-aspartate, an amino acid used in the laboratory). This receptor acts as an ion channel for Na^+, K^+, and Ca^{++} ions and may be important in both development and learning and memory.

Activation of NMDA receptors appears to lead to the production of the newly discovered neurotransmitter, *nitric oxide*. The calcium which enters the cell following binding of glutamate to the NMDA receptor binds to the regulatory protein calmodulin, and activates the enzyme nitric oxide synthase. This leads to the production of nitric oxide, a reactive neurotransmitter which has a half life of only a few seconds. The nitric oxide diffuses into nearby neurons, binding to and activating the enzyme *guanylyl cyclase*, which catalyzes the formation of the second messenger *cyclic GMP*. Interestingly, inhibitors of nitric oxide synthase prevent NMDA-induced neurotoxicity.

This "excitotoxicity" such as is produced by glutamate may be involved in development of neurodegenerative disorders such as Huntington's disease and Alzheimer's disease. Exposure to the neurotoxin and animal procarcinogen cycasin, and to β-*N*-methylamino-*L*-alanine (*BMAA*) an excitatory amino acid found in cycad seed may be associated with development of the neurodegenerative disease amyotrophic lateral sclerosis-Parkinsonism-dementia on the island of Guam and parts of Japan and Indonesia. Oddly enough, neurons which contain nitric oxide synthase seem to be resistant to both NMDA-induced neurotoxicity AND to damage from strokes, Alzheimer's disease, and Huntington's disease!

Kainic acid, a glutamate agonist, probably acts in a similar manner to NMDA, but binds to a different subset of glutamate receptors. Damage produced by kainic acid resembles damage resulting from the inherited disorder *Huntington's disease*. A naturally occurring excitatory neurotoxin, *quinolinic acid*, may be involved in development of this genetic disorder.

Some neurotoxicants damage neurons in very specific areas of the brain. One example is the organometal *trimethyltin* (TMT), which kills neurons in the hippocampus (a region of the cerebrum) and surrounding areas. The hippocampus plays a role in acquisition of memories, and is also part of the *limbic system*, which is important in emotional response. Animals treated with trimethyltin show behavioral changes consistent with disruption of these functions: they are quite aggressive, and there is evidence that memory-related processes may also be affected.

Another specific neurotoxicant is *MPTP*, a contaminant of a synthetic heroin-like drug of abuse called MPPP. MPTP neurotoxicity in humans was first reported by a group of doctors in 1982 who traced the cause of puzzling Parkinson's disease-like symptoms in young adult patients to their exposure to MPTP. In *Parkinson's disease*, normally a disease of the elderly, neurons are gradually lost from an area of the midbrain called the *substantia nigra*. These dopamine-producing neurons release their neurotransmitter onto neurons in the *basal ganglia* (an area of the brain important in movement), and the dopamine deficiency that accompanies their loss results in symptoms including tremor, slow movement, and rigidity.

MPTP not only produces symptoms that are virtually identical to Parkinson's disease, but also appears to act in the same manner, killing cells in the substantia nigra. Because of its lipid solubility, MPTP enters the brain easily where it accumulates in the affected neurons. MPTP itself is not neurotoxic but it is metabolized by the enzyme MAO (which breaks down catecholamines) to form a toxic derivative, MPP^+. MPP^+ may contribute to cell damage through production of free radicals, or perhaps through inhibition of mitochondrial enzymes. Further research on MPTP may help the search for causes and treatment of Parkinson's disease. Some scientists hypothesize that the cause of Parkinson's disease might be environmental. MPTP is structurally quite similar to the herbicide *paraquat*, and at least one intriguing study has found a higher incidence of Parkinson's disease among those with high pesticide exposures.

Other toxicants such as *carbon disulfide* also act in part through destruction of CNS neurons.

MERCURY
see also:

OTHER NEUROTOXICANTS

There are many other neurotoxicants, several with mechanisms of action that are not fully understood. Heavy metals such as *organic and inorganic mer-*

cury compounds are neurotoxic. Occupational exposure to inorganic mercury in the hat industry several hundred years ago gave rise to the phrase "mad as a hatter" as well as serving as inspiration for the character of the Mad Hatter in Lewis Carroll's *Alice's Adventures in Wonderland.* Symptoms of mercury poisoning may include depression, moodiness, insom-

---

LEAD
see also:

---

nia, and confusion, as well as tremors. Exposure to organic mercury compounds such as methylmercury produces tremors, motor dysfunction, and sensory disturbances. A major case of human exposure to methylmercury occurred in Minamata Japan, and is discussed elsewhere in this book.

Another neurotoxic metal is *lead.* Aside from the peripheral effects already discussed, lead also has effects on the central nervous system. These effects are collectively termed *lead encephalopathy.* Lead produces excitation of the central nervous system, leading to insomnia, restlessness, irritability, and convulsions. Children are more susceptible than adults, and recovery is in general not complete.

Another example of a class of neurotoxicants is the *halogenated hydrocarbon solvents.* Because of their lipid solubility they enter the central nervous system easily. Exposure to these solvents typically produces disorientation, euphoria, and confusion—symptoms that are reversible upon termination of exposure. Higher concentrations can lead to death, usually from depression of brain areas that stimulate respiration.

Other solvents, including

HALOGENATED HYDROCARBON SOLVENTS
see also:

---

aromatic solvents (benzene, toluene), and *alcohols* have similar effects. Several of these toxicants pose significant hazards as drugs of abuse. Toluene, for example, is used as a solvent in paints, glues, and other household products, and may be abused by "glue sniffers." Ethanol is perhaps the most widely used drug in this country. Ethanol is a central nervous system depressant, producing depression of inhibitions and mild euphoria at low levels (blood alcohol levels of 0.1%), but leading to impairment of reflexes, decreased sensory function, and loss of consciousness, coma, and even death at high levels (0.4 to 0.5%). The mechanism by which alcohol and other solvents produce their effects is not known, but probably involves actions on membranes and membrane fluidity.

EFFECTS ON SPECIAL SENSORY ORGANS

Many toxicants which affect peripheral neurons can indirectly affect sensory function, but there are some toxicants which affect specialized sensory organs such as the eye or ear directly. *Methanol*, for example, produces edema specifically in the optic nerve, leading to blindness (this is the origin of the phrase "blind drunk"). Some *excitatory amino acid neurotransmitters*, in addition to their other effects, damage cells in the retina. Finally, a number of compounds including *2,4-DNP*, *corticosteroids*, and *naphthalene* can produce reductions in transparency of the lens, commonly known as *cataracts*.

A few chemicals directly affect the ear. High doses of the antibiotic *streptomycin* can produce dizziness and hearing loss as a result of damage to the *vestibular apparatus* (which regulates balance) and the *cochlea* (the organ in the inner ear that responds to pressure waves and sends sensory signals to the brain). (Excessive exposure to *noise*, of course, can also damage the cochlea and lead to significant hearing loss.) *Aspirin* may produce a temporary hearing impairment characterized by tinnitus (ringing of the ears).

DEVELOPMENTAL EFFECTS

The period during which the nervous system develops is quite long, extending from a few days postconception to well into the postnatal (after birth) period. Exposure to toxicants during this developmental period is likely to have quite different effects on an organism than exposure to the same toxicant after growth and development is complete. Developmental neurotoxicants and their effects are discussed in Chapter 6.

METHODS IN NEUROTOXICOLOGY

There are many different methods which are used to study effects of neurotoxicants. These techniques include both *in vitro* techniques involving isolated tissues or chemicals, and *in vivo* techniques involving the whole animal. Although it is impossible to produce here a comprehensive list of all neurotoxicological techniques, some representative approaches will be discussed.

One major technique used in neurotoxicology is the study of *behavior*. In *operant conditioning*, an animal is trained (in an apparatus called a Skinner box) to press a lever to obtain a reward. In *classical conditioning*, a stimulus called the conditioning stimulus is paired with another stimulus that evokes a response from an animal (in the classic example, Pavlov paired the ringing of a bell with the presentation of food which evoked the response of salivation). Eventually, presentation of the conditioning stimulus alone is sufficient to evoke the response. If toxicant-treated animals respond differently to these two types of conditioning than control animals do, it can be an indication that the toxicant has nervous system effects. Effects could be sensory (inability to sense a stimulus), motor (inability to press a bar), or integrative (effects on learning and/or memory).

Some behavioral tests are specially designed to detect sensory dysfunction. For example, the *acoustic startle chamber* is a box with speakers and a special pressure-sensitive platform. Sounds of different frequencies and intensities are played through the speakers, and the startle reflex of the animal is measured. A variation of this is the air puff startle, where instead of sound the stimulus is a puff of air.

Motor function, too, can be measured. The activity of an animal in a *maze* or on a flat open platform called an *open field* can be measured. The motor activity measured by these methods is called *exploratory behavior*. Other tests of motor ability and coordination include descent down a rope, ability to stay on a rotating rod, and tests of walking ability (which is sometimes measured by dipping the animals feet in ink and examining the footprints it leaves).

Finally, observation of various behaviors can be an important testing method. Neurotoxicants can cause alterations in feeding behavior, mating behavior, reproductive behavior, and other social behaviors.

On a physiological level, some studies focus on the measurement of electrical activity of neurons. An *electroencephalogram* (EEG) measures electrical activity of the brain by measuring the potential difference (voltage) between electrodes that are placed on the scalp in humans and sometimes directly onto the surface of the brain in experimental animals. *Sensory evoked potentials*, the changes in EEG resulting from sensory stimulation, can be measured. *Seizures* can also be chemically or electrically induced in experimental animals, and the EEG monitored. Toxicants may alter evoked potentials, or affect the induction and course of seizures.

Electrical conduction can also be studied on the biochemical level. One popular technique for studying effects of toxicants on ion channels in neurons is the *voltage clamp*. The voltage clamp uses an external energy source to maintain membrane potential at a desired value.

Other biochemical techniques focus on synaptic functions. *Receptors* can be isolated and characterized, and receptor binding by various molecules studied. Many other biochemical studies are possible, including studies of *neurotransmitter levels, enzyme activities, axonal transport*, etc.

Finally, recent advances in imaging techniques have allowed researchers to get a glimpse of the living, functioning brain. *Computerized tomography* (CT scan) equipment rotates an x-ray source around the head, shooting multiple narrow beams of x-rays through the brain and measuring the degree to which x-rays are absorbed at each point and ultimately reconstructing (by computer) an image of a brain slice.

Even more exciting is the *positron emission tomography* (PET) scan. Molecules such as glucose analogues (compounds which are structurally similar to glucose) or neurotransmitters are radioactively labeled with isotopes of oxygen, carbon, and nitrogen with short half-lives. As these isotopes decay, the positrons which are emitted combine almost immediately with electrons, thus releasing detectable gamma radiation. Detectors measure the radiation, and construct an image showing the location of the labelled molecules in the brain. Changes in PET images over time can indicate changes in brain activity.

REFERENCES

Asbury, A. K. and Brown, M. J., The evolution of structural changes in distal axonopathies, in *Experimental and Clinical Neurotoxicology*, Spencer, P. S. and Schaumburg, H. H., Eds., Williams and Wilkins, Baltimore, 1980, chap. 12.

Anthony, D. C. and Graham, D. G., Toxic responses of the nervous system, in *Casarett and Doull's Toxicology*, Amdur, M. O., Doull, J., and Klaassen, C. D., Eds., Pergamon Press, New York, 1991, chap. 13.

Bradbury, M. W. B., The structure and function of the blood-brain barrier, *Fed. Proc.*, 43, 186, 1984.

Brown, A. W., Aldridge, W. N., Street, B. W., and Verschoyle, R. D., The behavioral and neuropathologic sequelae of intoxication by trimethyltin compounds in the rat, *Am. J. Pathol.*, 97, 59, 1979.

Dunant, Y. and Israel, M., The release of acetylcholine, *Sci. Am.*, 252, 58, 1985.

Gilman, A. G., Goodman, L. S., and Gilman, A., *Goodman and Gilman's The Pharmacological Basis of Therapeutics*, Macmillan, New York, 1980.

Goldstein, G. W. and Betz, A. L., The blood-brain barrier, *Sci. Am.*, 255, 74, 1986.

Griffin, J. W. and Price, D. L., Proximal axonopathies induced by toxic chemicals, in *Experimental and Clinical Neurotoxicology*, Spencer, P. S. and Schaumburg, H. H., Eds., Williams and Wilkins, Baltimore, 1980, chap. 11.

Jacobs, J. M., Vascular permeability and neural injury, in *Experimental and Clinical Neurotoxicology*, Spencer, P. S. and Schaumburg, H. H., Eds., Williams and Wilkins, Baltimore, 1980, chap. 8.

Lewin, R., Parkinson's disease: an environmental cause?, *Science*, 229, 257, 1985.

Lowndes, H. E. and Baker, T., Toxic site of action in distal axonopathies, in *Experimental and Clinical Neurotoxicology*, Spencer, P. S. and Schaumburg, H. H., Eds., Williams and Wilkins, Baltimore, 1980, chap. 13.

Morell, P. and Norton, W. T., Myelin, *Sci. Am.*, 242, 88, 1980.

Narahashi, T., Nerve membrane as a target of environmental toxicants, in *Experimental and Clinical Neurotoxicology*, Spencer, P. S. and Schaumburg, H. H., Eds., Williams and Wilkins, Baltimore, 1980, chap. 16.

Norton, S., Methods in behavioral neurotoxicology, in *Principles and Methods of Toxicology*, Hayes, A. W., Ed., Raven Press, New York, 1982, chap. 11.

Norton, S., Toxic responses of the central nervous system, in *Casarett and Doull's Toxicology*, Klaassen, C. D., Amdur, M. O., and Doull, J., Eds., Macmillan, New York, 1986, chap. 13.

Olney, J. W., Excitotoxic mechanisms of neurotoxicity, in *Experimental and Clinical Neurotoxicology*, Spencer, P. S. and Schaumburg, H. H., Eds., Williams and Wilkins, Baltimore, 1980, chap. 19.

Potts, A. M., Toxic responses of the eye, in *Casarett and Doull's Toxicology*, Amdur, M. O., Doull, J., and Klaassen, C. D., Eds., Pergamon Press, New York, 1991, chap. 17.

Prosen, C. A. and Stebbins, W. C., Ototoxicity, in *Experimental and Clinical Neurotoxicology*, Spencer, P. S. and Schaumburg, H. H., Eds., Williams and Wilkins, Baltimore, 1980, chap. 5.

Rasminsky, M., Physiological consequences of demyelination, in *Experimental and Clinical Neurotoxicology*, Spencer, P. S. and Schaumburg, H. H., Eds., Williams and Wilkins, Baltimore, 1980, chap. 18.

Russell, F. E., Toxic effects of animal toxins, in *Casarett and Doull's Toxicology*, Klaassen, C. D., Amdur, M. O., and Doull, J., Eds., Macmillan, New York, 1986, chap. 22.

Schwartz, J. H., Axonal transport: components, mechanisms, and specificity, *Annu. Rev. Neurosci.*, 2, 467, 1979.

Schwartz, J. H., The transport of substances in nerve cells, *Sci. Am.*, 242, 152, 1980.

Shankland, D. L., Neurotoxic action of chlorinated hydrocarbon insecticides, *Neurobehav. Toxicol. Teratol.*, 4, 805, 1982.

Shepherd, G. M., *Neurobiology*, Oxford University Press, New York, 1988.

Simpson, L. L., Molecular pharmacology of botulinum toxin and tetanus toxin, *Annu. Rev. Pharmacol. Toxicol.*, 26, 427, 1986.

Snyder, S. H. and Bredt, D. S., Biological roles of nitric oxide, *Sci. Am.*, May, 1992, 68.

Strichartz, G., Rando, T., and Wang, G. K., An integrated view of the molecular toxicology of sodium channel gating in excitable cells, *Annu. Rev. Neurosci.*, 10, 237, 1987.

Ter-Pogossian, M. M., Raichle, M. E., and Sobel, B. E., Positron emission tomography, *Sci. Am.*, 243, 171, 1980.

Wu, C. H. and Narahashi, T., Mechanism of action of novel marine neurotoxins on ion channels, *Annu. Rev. Pharmacol. Toxicol.*, 28, 141, 1988.

10 HEPATIC TOXICOLOGY

FUNCTION OF THE LIVER

The liver is an organ with an important role in many metabolic processes. Nutrient-containing blood from the gastrointestinal tract travels first to the liver (via the portal vein), where nutrients such as carbohydrates, lipids, and vitamins can be removed and stored until needed. Liver cells are also capable of metabolism of carbohydrates, lipids, and proteins.

The liver also synthesizes and secretes *bile*, which contains water, ions, lipids (cholesterol derivatives known as *bile salts*), and *bile pigments* (such as bilirubin). Bile is stored in the gall bladder and secreted into the small intestine where it plays an important role in both absorption and excretion.

The liver is, of course, also a site where significant xenobiotic metabolism occurs. This means that hepatocytes are at risk for exposure to the toxic bioactivated metabolites which result from the metabolism of some toxicants. The direct routing of blood to the liver from the gastrointestinal tract from which ingested xenobiotics are absorbed, as well as the tendency for some compounds to undergo enterohepatic cycling (repeated reabsorption from bile and return to the liver), also increase the vulnerability of liver cells to assault from toxicants.

ANATOMY AND PHYSIOLOGY OF THE LIVER

The liver is a large organ located in the upper abdomen and is separated in humans into two major and two minor *lobes* (Figure 1). Blood enters the liver from two sources: the *hepatic artery* (brings blood from the systemic circulation), and the *portal vein* (brings blood directly from the gastrointestinal tract). Blood exits the liver via the *hepatic vein*, and bile passes out through the *hepatic duct* and then either through the *common bile duct* to the small intestine, or through the *cystic duct* to the *gall bladder* for storage.

The cells in the liver are arranged in distinctive hexagonal patterns which have been called *lobules* (Figure 2). Epithelial cells called *hepatocytes* appear to

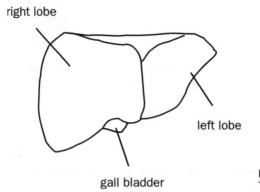

right lobe

left lobe

gall bladder

Figure 1
The liver.

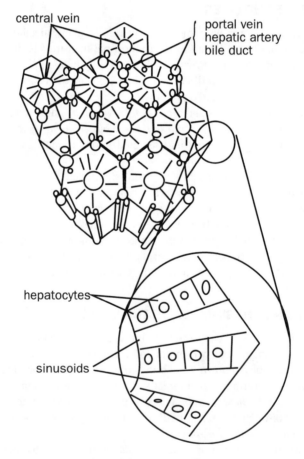

central vein

portal vein
hepatic artery
bile duct

hepatocytes

sinusoids

Figure 2   The hepatic lobule.

radiate outward from a *central vein* (which is actually a branch of the hepatic vein). The columns of hepatocytes have between them channels called *sinusoids* which are lined with highly permeable endothelial cells and which also contain phagocytic cells called *Kupffer cells*. Three other vessels are found at each of the outer corners of the hexagon (the *portal area*): a branch of the portal vein, a branch of the hepatic artery, and a bile duct. Blood flows in through the branches of the hepatic artery and portal vein, passes through the sinusoids, and flows out through the central vein. Bile is manufactured in the hepatocytes, and flows out through *bile canaliculi* (located between adjacent hepatocytes) to the bile ducts.

Studies have shown, though, that lobules are not self-contained functional units. Each hepatic artery/portal vein pair supplies blood not to just one lobule, but to a region of cells which overlaps two or more lobules. This area has been termed an *acinus* (Figure 3). The more current, and functionally accurate picture of the liver focuses on acini rather than lobules. The characteristics of hepatocytes vary with their location in the acinus. Three acinar zones have been defined, based on the distance from the blood-supplying vessels. Cells in zone 1 show a high activity of enzymes involved in respiration; zone 1 also seems to be the site where regeneration and replacement of liver cells begins (the new cells then migrate outward through

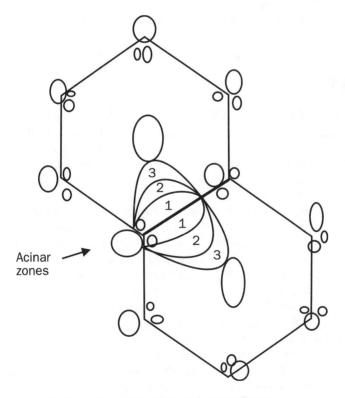

Figure 3   The hepatic acinus and surrounding zones.

zones 2 and 3). Cells in zone 3, on the other hand, show high cytochrome P450 activity. An alternative descriptive scheme (based on the earlier lobule model) describes cells as being *centrilobular* (near the central vein, roughly corresponding to zone 3), *periportal* (near the portal area, corresponding to parts of zones 1, 2, and 3), or *midzonal* (along the edge between lobules, corresponding to the remainder of zone 1).

One main function of the liver is, of course, to assist in the absorption, metabolism, and storage of nutrients. When blood glucose levels rise (following a meal, for example), hepatocytes convert glucose to either glycogen or fats for storage. Conversely, when blood glucose levels fall, hepatocytes breakdown glycogen to release glucose into the bloodstream, and can also convert amino acids and other sugars into glucose. Bile helps breakdown fat globules in the small intestine, aiding the work of digestive enzymes. Hepatocytes can breakdown, synthesize, and store fats, and can package lipids together with proteins to form the lipoproteins which transport lipids through the bloodstream to other cells. Finally, hepatocytes play a critical role in protein metabolism by modifying and breaking down amino acids, converting ammonia into urea (for excretion in the urine), and synthesizing plasma proteins.

The liver also is important in maintenance of proper blood volume and composition. The liver stores blood, and phagocytizes damaged red blood cells. Bile serves as a vehicle for the disposal of bilirubin—a waste product of hemoglobin breakdown.

XENOBIOTIC METABOLISM
see also:
Biotransformation   *Ch. 3, p. 21*

The role of the liver in xenobiotic metabolism and excretion of toxicants is discussed in detail in Chapter 3, so only the basics will be reviewed here. Many hepatocytes contain enzyme systems capable of chemically altering toxic compounds, usually to a less toxic form. There are two basic types of metabolic alterations which can occur, and these are usually referred to as Phase I and Phase II reactions.

Phase I reactions involve oxidation or hydrolysis (or sometimes even reduction) of the compound, and are carried out by an enzyme system called the *cytochrome P450 system* or by various hydrolases. This system involves a number of different enzymes, including multiple forms of cytochrome P450 itself. Some of these forms are involved in metabolism of steroids and other endogenous compounds, whereas others metabolize xenobiotics. Two of the major groups of P450 enzymes involved in xenobiotic metabolism are the group of enzymes which is inducible by phenobarbital, and the group which is inducible by polycyclic aromatic hydrocarbons (commonly referred to as cytochrome P448).

Phase II reactions involve conjugation of the toxicant (or often a metabolite resulting from a Phase I reaction) with some other molecule. Generally, this action increases the size and water solubility of the toxicant, leading to enhanced excretion.

TYPES OF TOXICANT-INDUCED LIVER INJURY

Fatty Liver

Since the liver is the site of synthesis, storage, and release of lipids, it stands to reason that interference with these processes could lead to an accumulation of fats in the liver itself. Acute exposure to compounds such as *carbon tetrachloride*, *ethionine*, and *tetracycline* (an antibiotic) or chronic exposure to ethanol can block the secretion of a type of lipid called triglycerides, leading to the development of what is commonly called a "fatty liver" where anywhere from 5 to 50% of the liver's weight is fat.

CARBON TETRACHLORIDE	
see also:	
Biotransformation	*Ch. 3, p. 32*
Cardiovascular	
toxicology	*Ch. 8, p. 106*
Neurotoxicology	*Ch. 9, p. 143*
Hepatotoxicology	*Ch. 10, p. 154, 156*
Renal toxicology	*Ch. 10, pp. 166*
Halogenated	
hydrocarbons	*Appendix, p. 238*

The liver can take free fatty acids and by combining them with glycerol, can synthesize triglycerides. These triglycerides are then combined with phospholipids, cholesterol, and proteins to form *very low density lipoproteins* (*VLDLs*). VLDLs then enter the bloodstream, carrying triglycerides to other cells. The mechanisms by which fatty liver is produced are not completely clear but the most likely hypotheses involve inhibition of VLDL synthesis, perhaps through inhibition of the synthesis of the protein component (in the case of ethionine and carbon tetrachloride) or interference with the joining of the lipids and protein together. Defects in lipid metabolism might also be involved. For example, there is some experimental evidence that exposure to ethanol may lead to an increase in fatty acid synthesis, which may then contribute to a large increase in triglyceride synthesis. Also, inhibition of synthesis of the phospholipid component of VLDL could occur. Other evidence has indicated that inhibition of release of the lipoprotein may be a factor. Interestingly enough, the presence of the excess fat in the liver does not necessarily affect the functioning of the hepatocytes.

Liver Necrosis

A number of compounds have been reported to cause hepatic *necrosis*, or cell death. Necrosis of hepatocytes is characterized by accumulation of vacuoles in the cytoplasm, damage to endoplasmic reticulum, swelling of mitochondria, destruction of the nucleus, and disruption of the plasma membrane. Necrosis is often described as being either focal (confined to a limited area), zonal, diffuse, or massive, and its location is frequently described using the descriptive terms (introduced earlier) centrilobular, midzonal, or periportal.

One possible mechanism of injury to hepatocytes is lipid peroxidation.

LIPID PEROXIDATION
see also:

CARBON TETRACHLORIDE
see also:

Compounds such as *carbon tetrachloride* are metabolized by cytochrome P450 to form free radicals, reactive metabolites which can bind to and damage macromolecules. Unsaturated fatty acids in membranes are particularly vulnerable to attack by free radicals. Carbon tetrachloride exposure has been shown to produce damage to membranes including smooth and rough endoplasmic reticulum, thus reducing xenobiotic-metabolizing ability as well as reducing protein synthesis. In fact a small initial dose of carbon tetrachloride protects against injury from a later larger dose, probably by destroying P450 and limiting the ability of the liver to bioactivate the later dose. Further evidence that carbon tetrachloride produces lipid peroxidation is found in the production of molecules called conjugated dienes, which are frequently used to monitor the occurrence of lipid peroxidation. Administration of antioxidants (to reduce or prevent lipid peroxidation) prevented some but not all toxic effects of carbon tetrachloride, indicating that even though lipid peroxidation is a factor, other mechanisms are probably also involved. Endogenous enzymes such as superoxide dismutase may play a role in limiting peroxidation *in vivo*.

Carbon tetrachloride is not the only compound to be converted to an active, toxic metabolite by cytochrome P450. *Chloroform, bromobenzene*, and many other *halogenated hydrocarbons* are also metabolized by P450 to reactive compounds. *Acetaminophen*, a common over-the-counter analgesic, is oxidized to form a toxic metabolite capable of covalent binding to hepatic proteins and other cellular constituents. Because these toxicants depend on bioactivation to produce their effects, the necrosis which they produce tends to be centrilobular (located in zone 3). This area, as you may recall, is where the greatest P450 activity is located. Also, the toxicity of these compounds can be potentiated by compounds which induce cytochrome P450 activity. Ethanol, for example, potentiates the effects of carbon tetrachloride and other halogenated hydrocarbons, probably through effects on P450. The ability of the liver to perform Phase II reactions is also a significant factor in determining the toxicity of these compounds. For example, many of the reactive metabolites produced in Phase I undergo binding to glutathione and other Phase II cofactors, thus limiting binding to cellular sites. Thus, competition of other toxicants for binding to cofactors or dietary depletion of cofactors may potentiate the toxicity of these compounds.

Which of the many effects of these toxicants is actually responsible for the death of the cell is a subject of considerable debate. It

---

CELL DEATH
see also:
   Cellular sites of action   *Ch. 4, p. 37*

---

is probably not inhibition of protein synthesis, because toxicants such as ethionine can do this for hours without killing the cell. Damage to mitochondria has also been suggested as the lethal trigger, but as with inhibition of protein synthesis, ATP depletion can be observed without necrosis. Many theories point to effects on calcium homeostasis, since increased intercellular calcium levels frequently accompany cell death, and damage to membranes (such as the endoplasmic reticulum or mitochondrial membrane) could lead to release of sequestered calcium. Entry of external calcium into the cell through a damaged plasma membrane may or may not be involved, as studies have indicated that an external pool of calcium is not necessary to produce necrosis. It is difficult, however, to determine if the increase in calcium actually causes the death of the cell, or if it is a result of it.

Cirrhosis

Chronic exposure to hepatotoxicants can lead to a condition called *cirrhosis*. A combination of damage to hepatocytes and inadequate regeneration leads to increased activity of fibroblasts, and accumulation of collagen in the liver. This results in not only a net loss of functioning hepatocytes, but also in a significant disruption of blood flow in the liver. Chronic exposure to *ethanol* is a leading cause of cirrhosis in humans, but the mechanism underlying the effect is the subject of considerable debate. Malnutrition fre-

---

ETHANOL
see also:
   Reproductive toxicology   *Ch. 6, p. 82*
   Neurotoxicology   *Ch. 9, p. 143*
   Ethanol   *Appendix, p. 237*

---

quently accompanies alcoholism, and some investigators hypothesize that it is this factor, rather than the alcohol, which causes the cirrhosis. Evidence has been presented showing that rats who are maintained on an adequate diet can be exposed to ethanol without developing cirrhosis, but other studies have indicated that monkeys develop precirrhotic changes with exposure to ethanol even if no nutritional deficiencies develop.

Miscellaneous Effects

Exposure to some toxicants produces *cholestasis*, or stoppage of bile flow. This results in the development of *jaundice*, a condition characterized by a yellowish discoloration of the eyes and skin (resulting from the buildup of bile pigments such as bilirubin). This occurs in humans primarily following administration of drugs such as steroids, phenothiazines, and tricyclic antidepressants. The mechanism for this effect is not clear. Exposure to other toxicants (such as the anesthetic *halothane*) can cause a condition resembling viral *hepatitis*, with headache, nausea, vomiting, dizziness, and jaundice. This effect may be caused at least in part by a reaction of the immune system to the drug.

Carcinogenesis

Many hepatotoxicants, including carbon tetrachloride and chloroform have also been shown to be hepatic carcinogens in laboratory animals. Another group of potential hepatic carcinogens are the *aflatoxins*, toxins produced by a fungus which grows on grain and other foods. Aflatoxin B_1, for example, is metabolized by cytochrome P450 to a reactive epoxide, which then can bind to DNA. Some *PCBs* may also be hepatic carcinogens. The most well known human hepatic carcinogen is probably *vinyl chloride* a chemical used in the manufacture of polyvinyl chloride (PVC). Its carcinogenic potential was discovered when it became clear that workers exposed to vinyl chloride were developing an unusually large number of cases of the relatively rare type of liver cancer known as *angiosarcoma*.

CARBON TETRACHLORIDE
see also:

Biotransformation	***Ch. 3, p. 32***
Cardiovascular	
toxicology	***Ch. 8, p. 106***
Neurotoxicology	***Ch. 9, p. 143***
Hepatotoxicology	**Ch. 10, pp. 153, 154**
Renal toxicology	***Ch. 11, p. 166***
Halogenated	
hydrocarbons	***Appendix, p. 238***

EVALUATING LIVER INJURY

Several methods, both clinical and experimental, are used to test for injury to the liver. *Serum enzyme tests* look for activity of enzymes in the blood which are normally found in hepatic cells. Increased serum activities of these enzymes may indicate damage to hepatocytes, and subsequent leakage of the enzymes. Enzymes which are typically assessed may include aminotransferases such as serum glutamic-oxaloacetic transaminase (*SGOT*) and serum glutamic-pyruvic transaminase (*SGPT*), serum alkaline phosphatase (AP), serum lactate dehydrogenase (*LDH*), and many others. Some of these enzymes are more specific for liver injury than others (which may be elevated when other tissues are injured, also). On the other hand, some are specific enough not only to indicate liver injury, but to aid in diagnosing the type of injury.

REFERENCES

James, R. C., Hepatotoxicity: toxic effects in the liver, in *Industrial Toxicology*, Williams, P. L. and Burson, J. L., Eds., Van Nostrand Reinhold, New York, 1985, chap. 5.

Kulkarni, A. P. and Hodgson, E., Hepatotoxicity, in *Introduction to Biochemical Toxicology*, Hodgson, E. and Guthrie, F. E., Eds., Elsevier, New York, 1980, chap. 18.

Mehendale, H. M., Hepatotoxicity, in *Handbook of Toxicology*, Haley, T. J. and Berndt, W. O. Eds., Hemisphere, Washington, 1987, chap. 4.

Plaa, G. L., Toxic responses of the liver, in *Casarett and Doull's Toxicology*, Amdur, M. O., Doull, J., and Klaassen, C. D., Eds., Pergamon Press, New York, 1991, chap. 10.

Plaa, G. L. and Hewitt, W. R., Detection and evaluation of chemically induced liver injury, in *Principles and Methods of Toxicology*, Hayes, A. W., Ed., Raven Press, New York, 1989, chap. 20.

Pransky, G., Hepatic disorders, in *Occupational Health*, Levy, B. S. and Wegman, D. H., Eds., Little, Brown, and Company, Boston, 1983, chap. 25.

Sipes, I. G. and Gandolfi, A. J., Biotransformation of toxicants, in *Casarett and Doull's Toxicology*, Amdur, M. O., Doull, J., and Klaassen, C. D., Eds., Pergamon Press, New York, 1991, chap. 12.

11   RENAL TOXICOLOGY

FUNCTION OF THE KIDNEYS

The major functions of the kidneys are to *excrete waste* (including soluble xenobiotics and conjugates) from the blood through formation of urine, and to *regulate body levels of water and salts* such as potassium and sodium. In addition, hormones and enzymes produced by the kidney are important in the *regulation of blood pressure, pH levels, calcium metabolism, and the production of red blood cells.*

ANATOMY AND PHYSIOLOGY OF THE KIDNEYS

The kidneys are found in the abdominal area, near the posterior wall. The structure of a kidney is defined by several morphological features (Figure 1). Each kidney is covered by an outer *capsule*. Underneath the capsule is a layer of tissue called the *cortex*, and an inner zone known as the *medulla*. Blood enters the kidney through the *renal artery*, and leaves via the *renal vein*. The cortex receives the bulk of the blood flow to the kidney, and has a much higher rate of oxygen utilization than the medulla. (As we will see, most of the energy-intensive processes in the kidney occur in the cortex.) Urine leaving the kidney passes through the renal *pelvis* and out the *ureter*.

The functional unit of the kidney is the *nephron* (Figure 2), with each kidney containing around a million nearly identical nephrons. Each nephron is composed of a *glomerulus* surrounded by a structure called *Bowman's Capsule*, and a tubule consisting of a *proximal* portion, a loop (*Loop of Henle*), a *distal* portion, and a *collecting duct*. The glomerular portion of every nephron is located in the cortex, but while the tubules of some nephrons are found only in the cortex, the tubules of nephrons located deep in the cortex extend into the medulla.

Fluid from the blood is filtered at the glomerulus, and then passes into the tubule. In the proximal tubule, many substances in the filtrate are reabsorbed by

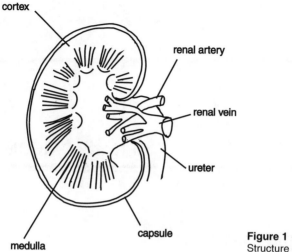

cortex

renal artery

renal vein

ureter

capsule

medulla

Figure 1
Structure of the kidney.

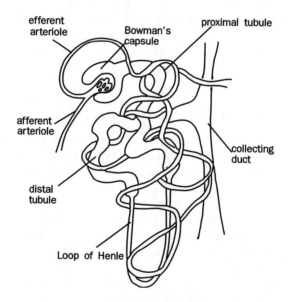

efferent
arteriole

Bowman's
capsule

proximal tubule

afferent
arteriole

collecting
duct

distal
tubule

Loop of Henle

Figure 2   The nephron.

the epithelial cells lining the tubule. In addition, some substances which were not filtered are secreted by the proximal tubule cells into the filtrate. The filtrate is further concentrated in the remaining portions of the tubule, and eventually is excreted as urine.

EFFECTS OF TOXICANTS ON THE KIDNEY—GENERAL PRINCIPLES

Toxicant-induced damage to the kidney may be mild or severe, reversible or permanent, depending on the toxic agent and the dose. The kidney is particularly susceptible to the effects of toxicants for several reasons. First, blood flow to the kidneys is high (25% of cardiac output), so blood-borne toxicants will be delivered to the kidneys in large quantities. Second, as the kidney removes salts, water, and other substances from the filtrate through the process of reabsorption, any toxicant that is not reabsorbed may become highly concentrated in the remaining filtrate. Finally, even if a toxicant *is* reabsorbed, it still may accumulate to high concentrations within the tubule cells themselves. Thus, kidney tubule cells may be exposed to concentrations of a toxicant which are many times higher than the concentration of that toxicant in the plasma. In addition, many cells have cytochrome P450 activity, so if bioactivation of a toxicant occurs, those cells may be affected.

DAMAGE TO THE GLOMERULUS

One site at which nephrotoxicants may act is the glomerulus (shown in Figure 3). The glomerulus itself is a network of capillaries arising from an *afferent arteriole*, a branch of the renal artery. The walls of the glomerular capillaries are very porous. Blood enters the glomerulus at relatively high pressure (around 60 mm Hg). This pressure, which is regulated in part by specialized cells of the afferent arteriole called juxtaglomerular cells, forces blood fluids out of the pores, across a basement membrane and through filtration slits between the podocytes (the epithelial cells that makeup Bowman's Capsule). The capillaries reunite upon exiting Bowman's Capsule, forming an *efferent arteriole* which then branches into a second network of capillaries around the tubule. Efferent arterioles eventually empty into the renal vein.

Thus, the glomerulus acts as a filter, allowing the passage of 20 to 40% of plasma fluids and small molecules into Bowman's Capsule, but retaining blood cells and most plasma proteins (which are too large to fit through the filter) in the bloodstream. In addition to molecular size, net electrical charge of a molecule affects filtration, with neutral molecules more likely to pass through the glomerular membrane which is itself negatively charged. In a normal person, a total of around 125 ml of fluid per minute is filtered by the two kidneys. This number is called the *glomerular filtration rate*, or *GFR*.

Toxicants may increase permeability of the glomerulus, resulting in proteinuria, the leakage of large molecular weight proteins into the filtrate, and thus into the urine. Some toxicants can reduce the negative charge of the glomerular membrane and can lead to the excretion of large anions. Other toxicants may damage podocytes, increasing filtration slit size. One compound which produces both these effects is the antibiotic *puromycin*.

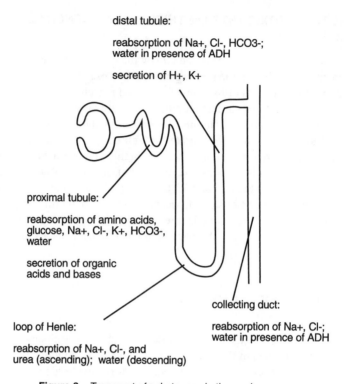

distal tubule:

reabsorption of Na+, Cl-, HCO3-;
water in presence of ADH

secretion of H+, K+

proximal tubule:

reabsorption of amino acids,
glucose, Na+, Cl-, K+, HCO3-,
water

secretion of organic
acids and bases

collecting duct:

loop of Henle:

reabsorption of Na+, Cl-, and
urea (ascending); water (descending)

reabsorption of Na+, Cl-;
water in presence of ADH

Figure 3   Transport of substances in the nephron.

DAMAGE TO THE PROXIMAL TUBULE

As the filtrate traverses the length of the tubule, several processes occur in various areas (Figure 4). The first part of the tubule is called the *proximal tubule* and is perhaps the major site of action for nephrotoxicants. The proximal tubule has two sections: a twisted or *convoluted* section, and a straight section or *pars recta*. The cells lining the proximal tubule have a *tubular* or *luminal* side facing into the lumen of the tubule (with a convoluted surface called a *brush border*), and a *peritubular* side facing out toward the efferent capillaries. These cells perform the important function of *reabsorption* of 60 to 80% of the filtrate constituents. The maximum rate of reabsorption for a substance is called its *tubular maximum* or T_{max}. Among the substances which are reabsorbed in the proximal tubule are:

1. Electrolytes: Na^+ in the form of NaCl or $NaHCO_3$ is reabsorbed by an active transport mechanism. The sodium diffuses into the proximal tubule cell across the tubular membrane, then is actively pumped out across the peritubular membrane where it is reabsorbed into the capillaries of the efferent arterioles (Figure 4). K^+ on the other hand, is actively pumped into the cell across the

to proximal tubule

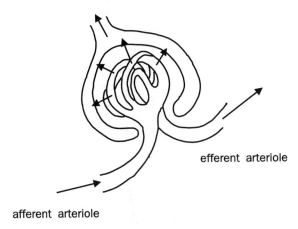

efferent arteriole

afferent arteriole

Figure 4   The glomerulus.

tubular membrane. Other ions such as potassium, magnesium, calcium, phosphates, and sulfates are also reabsorbed. Bicarbonate (HCO_{3-}) is also reabsorbed, but indirectly. The reabsorption of this important buffer is tied to the secretion of H^+, and is described later.

2. Glucose: Glucose is reabsorbed, perhaps through a cotransport mechanism with sodium. Normally, all glucose in the filtrate is reabsorbed. This mechanism can be saturated, though, if blood glucose levels are high enough (for example as a result of diabetes).

3. Amino Acids: Many amino acids are reabsorbed, some more effectively than others. It is probable that several different mechanisms are active in this pH-sensitive process.

Other substances which are reabsorbed include ascorbic acid, and to some extent urea and uric acid. Water is not actively reabsorbed, but is pulled osmotically along with electrolytes. Reabsorption in the proximal tubule is isosmotic: Although volume of the filtrate decreases, its osmolality (a measure of the concentration of dissolved particles in a solution) remains the same.

Another important process also occurs in the proximal tubule: the process of *secretion*. During the process of secretion, substances which remain in the bloodstream and are not filtered are pumped into the tubular lumen by the proximal tubule cells. There appear to be two major secretory transport systems: one for organic anions [substances such as *p*-aminohippurate (PAH) or the antibiotic penicillin], and one for organic cations [such as tetraethylammonium (TEA) or *N*-methylnicotinamide (NMN)]. Some electrolytes are secreted, as well. H^+, for example, is secreted as part of the process of maintaining the proper pH balance in the body. The secreted H^+ then combines with HCO_{3-} to

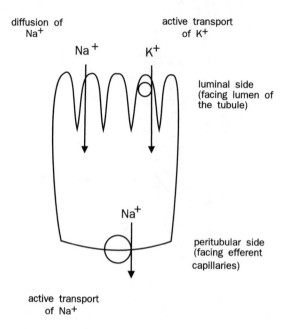

Figure 5   Transport of sodium and potassium in the proximal tubule cells.

form H_2CO_3, which then breaks down to $CO_2 + H_2O$. The CO_2 is reabsorbed and reforms H_2CO_3 within the cell. Thus the secretion of H^+ leads to the reabsorption of bicarbonate.

LIPID PEROXIDATION
see also:
   Cellular sites of action   Ch. 4, p. 51

Here in the proximal tubule, toxicants may damage proximal tubule cells, perhaps through formation of reactive oxygen species such as hydroxyl radicals. These species may then lead to membrane damage, including decreases in fluidity, effects on membrane-related proteins, or perhaps alterations in calcium homeostasis. Inhibition of reabsorption results, leading to appearance of glucose or amino acids in the urine (glycosuria, aminoaciduria). In addition, inhibition of salt reabsorption diminishes the coabsorption of water thus producing an increase in urine volume (polyuria). Eventually, though, severe proximal tubule damage leads to oliguria (decrease in urine flow) or anuria (stoppage of urine flow).

The mechanism by which oliguria and anuria are produced has been questioned. Some have hypothesized that sloughing off damaged proximal tubule cells obstructs the tubular lumen. It is also possible that increased leakiness in the proximal tubule may lead to loss of filtrate, or that vascular effects may also be involved, leading to a reduction in GFR.

One class of compounds which acts on the proximal tubule are the *heavy metals*. In addition to producing these functional indications of proximal cell dysfunction, microscopic examination of proximal cells following metal-induced nephrotoxicity reveals cell damage and *necrosis* (death).

Metals may act by binding to sulfhydryl groups on membranes and enzymes and disrupting their normal functions. (Administration of dithiothreitol, a sulfhydryl-containing mercury chelator was able to protect against mercury-induced renal toxicity.) As low a dosage as 1 mg/kg of a *mercuric salt*, for example, has been shown to

MERCURY
see also:
    Reproductive
      toxicology   *Ch. 6, p. 83*
    Neurotoxicology   *Ch. 9, p. 142*
    Water pollution   *Ch. 15, p. 222*
    Mercury   *Appendix, p. 239*

affect enzymes in the brush border of proximal tubule cells within minutes, with intracellular damage occurring several hours later. It is not clear, however, whether this intracellular damage, including effects on energy metabolism, is the primary cause of toxicity or merely a response to the initial membrane damage. Mercury toxicity may also involve effects on blood flow as well, with constriction of blood vessels causing a decrease in filtration as well as decreases in oxygen supply to renal tissues. The effects of organomercurials are similar, perhaps because they are metabolized to inorganic mercury.

Although heavy metals may be similar in many of their effects on proximal tubule function, some effects may differ (particularly at low doses). For example, mercury-induced damage is concentrated in that part of the proximal tubule where anion secretion occurs (the *pars recta*). Thus, organic anion secretion is particularly sensitive to mercury, while glucose reabsorption (which occurs in another section, the *convoluted*) is affected less. Low doses of *chromium*, on the other hand, produce marked inhibition of glucose reabsorption as a result of damage to the convoluted proximal tubule. In kidney slices *in vitro*, chromium actually stimulates anion secretion at low concentrations (10^{-6} M), although it inhibits secretion at higher concentrations (10^{-4} M).

Another metal which is a nephrotoxicant is *cadmium*. Cadmium accumulates in the kidney throughout life, with a half-life measured in tens of years in humans. Toxicity occurs when concentrations of cadmium

CADMIUM
see also:
    Reproductive toxicology   *Ch. 6, p. 75*
    Cardiovascular
      toxicology   *Ch. 8, p. 111*
    Water pollution   *Ch. 15, p. 222*
    Cadmium   *Appendix, p. 235*

in the kidney reach 200 μg/g kidney weight. The kidney contains cadmium- and zinc-binding proteins called metallothioneins. These stable, cytoplasmic proteins have low molecular weights and contain large amounts of cysteine. Exposure to cadmium, mercury, and other metals (but not zinc), causes an increase in renal metallothionein synthesis. In fact, studies have shown that pretreatment with low doses of cadmium can protect against damage from a later, larger dose. By binding to cadmium, metallothionein may prevent cadmium from binding to and damaging other cellular constituents, particularly in other organs. In the kidney, however, the cadmium-metallothionein complex itself can still damage kidney cells, particularly in later stages of chronic cadmium exposure.

HALOGENATED HYDROCARBON SOLVENTS

Certain *halogenated hydrocarbons* also affect the proximal tubule. As mentioned before, it is likely that these chemicals are metabolically activated by the cytochrome P450 activity found in the proximal tubule, producing free radicals which then damage membranes. Covalent binding of halogenated hydrocarbons such as bromobenzene and chloroform to renal proteins occurs in the proximal tubule cells, correlates with tissue damage, and appears to require some metabolic activation. In fact, differences in toxicity of these compounds between species may relate to quantitative and qualitative differences in renal P450 or glutathione concentrations. Additionally, inducers such as phenobarbital potentiate chloroform toxicity, while SH-containing compounds are protective.

Many antibiotics are nephrotoxic. For example, the *aminoglycosides* such as streptomycin, neomycin, and gentamicin produce damage to proximal tubule cells, perhaps through inhibition of phospholipases or through effects on mitochondrial function. *Cephalosporins* also are accumulated by and damage proximal tubule cells. Some analgesics also may bind to and damage membranes.

2,4,5-T

The herbicide *2,4,5-T*, while not directly nephrotoxic, can inhibit the organic anion secretion system, and at high enough concentrations may also inhibit cation secretion. PCBs, PBBs, and TCDD may indirectly influence nephrotoxicity by increasing renal P450 activity. Some compounds may produce what are called *obstructive uropathies. Ethylene glycol,* for example, is metabolized to oxalic acid, which is then deposited in the tubule lumen as calcium oxalate.

THE REMAINDER OF THE TUBULE

After leaving the proximal tubule, the filtrate continues into the *loop of Henle*. In the loop, distal tubule, and collecting duct, the filtrate becomes more concentrated through a process called a countercurrent mechanism. Chloride is actively reabsorbed in the ascending arm of the loop and moves into the area between the ascending and descending arm. Water must then leave the descending arm to compensate for the increase in osmolality in the area between the two arms. This creates a gradient, with increasing osmolality (electrolyte concentration) near the tip of the loop. Thus, the filtrate becomes more concentrated as it moves down the loop.

As the filtrate moves back up the ascending arm, the osmolality again begins to decrease. However, the impermeability of the ascending arm to water, along with further reabsorption of sodium and water in the distal tubule keeps the filtrate at a higher osmolality, and at a much lower volume (approximately 5 or 10% of the initial volume) than when it began its trip through the tubule.

The actual degree to which urine is concentrated depends on the permeability of the walls of the collecting duct. In the presence of *antidiuretic hormone* (ADH), the cells lining the duct become quite permeable, allowing water to leave the duct, and thus concentrating the urine. If no ADH is present, the cells will be impermeable to water, and little concentration will occur.

There are a few compounds which seem to exert their effects on these segments of the tubule. Many of them are pharmacological agents. Some *analgesics* (aspirin and phenacetin) produce damage to the medulla (which is where many of the loops and collecting ducts are located). This may be secondary to their effects on the blood vessels, however. (Aspirin inhibits synthesis of a class of compounds called prostaglandins which mediate vasodilation.)

Methoxyflurane, an anesthetic, may block the effects of ADH on the collecting duct (producing polyuria) as well as interfering with reabsorption of Na^+ and water in the proximal tubules. Metabolism may be necessary to produce these effects. *Tetracyclines*, a group of antibiotics, may also produce damage to the medulla.

MEASUREMENT OF KIDNEY FUNCTION *IN VIVO*

Many measurements of kidney function rely on the determination of the *renal clearance* of a chemical compound: $C = (U)(V)/(P)$, where C = clearance, U = concentration of the compound in the urine, V = urine flow, and P = concentration of the compound in the plasma. The physiological meaning of clearance is sometimes a somewhat difficult concept to grasp. It is *the volume of plasma which could be completely "cleared" of the substance in question in one minute*. Of course, because not all blood fluids are filtered, and due to the process of reabsorption, the kidneys do not always completely clear a substance in one pass through. Thus a clearance of 30 ml/min for a substance probably does not mean

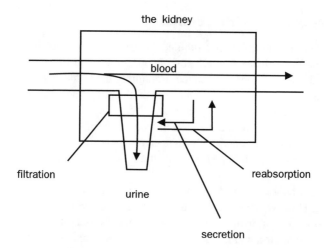

Figure 6 The concept of clearance. If a substance is completely cleared through secretion, clearance = renal plasma flow. If a substance is neither secreted nor reabsorbed, clearance is a reflection of glomerular filtration rate.

that an actual 30 ml of plasma is being completely cleared of the substance in one minute, but may instead mean that 120 ml of plasma is being cleared of one quarter of the substance in one minute. Each drug or chemical has its own clearance rate, which can be determined by experimentally measuring the three variables in the equation, if the compound follows first-order elimination kinetics.

Some substances, through filtration and secretion, *are* actually completely cleared from the plasma in one pass through the kidney. The clearance of one of these substances is then a measure of total plasma flow through the kidneys. This rate is called *renal plasma flow*, or RPF. The substance most commonly used to determine RPF is PAH.

If a substance is neither secreted nor reabsorbed, it will be totally removed only from the plasma filtrate, so its clearance will be a measure of the rate at which plasma is filtered. This is the glomerular filtration rate or GFR. One such substance is *inulin*, a polymer of fructose.

Along with monitoring RPF or GFR, kidney function can also be assessed by examining urine volume and constituents. Changes in urine volume, osmolality, or pH as well as presence of such normally absent substances as protein or glucose (proteinuria or glucosuria) may indicate kidney damage. Increases in levels of blood urea nitrogen (BUN) and plasma creatinine may also be used as indicators of kidney dysfunction. In addition, the presence in urine of specific enzymes (maltase, trehalase) normally found only in the brush border of proximal tubule cells may be an early indication of damage to these cells. One laboratory technique which has provided much useful information on kidney function is the *micropuncture* technique. In micropuncture, fluid can be collected from individual nephrons or capillaries within the kidney of an anesthetized animal (usually a rat or dog). Although this technique allows precise measurements of GFR, RPF, and filtrate volume and composition in a single nephron, the extensive training and experience required to perform the procedure hinder its widespread use.

MEASUREMENT OF KIDNEY FUNCTION *IN VITRO*

Isolated tissues are often used to study renal functions. Slices of renal cortex (which contain both proximal and distal tubule) will accumulate anions and cations, and are used to study the secretory process. Besides studying normal function, these studies are quite useful in toxicology. An animal may either be dosed with a toxicant prior to preparation of a kidney slice, or the toxicant may be added directly to the slice and its effects on these transport processes studied. Slices will also accumulate glucose, a process which appears to be related to reabsorption *in vivo* (rather than secretion as in the case of organic anions and cations).

Other techniques used to study renal function *in vitro* include the isolated perfused tubule technique. A segment of a nephron must be dissected out, perfused with fluid, and its function monitored. As with micropuncture, this is a sophisticated and difficult technique and thus not widely used.

REFERENCES

Berndt, W. O., Renal toxicology, in *Handbook of Toxicology*, Haley, T. J. and Berndt, W. O. Eds., Hemisphere Publishing Corporation, Washington, 1987, chap.

Berndt, W. O., Renal methods in toxicology, in *Principles and Methods in Toxicology*, Hayes, A. W., Ed., Raven Press, New York, 1982, chap.

Berndt, W. O., Effects of toxic chemicals on renal transport processes, *Fed. Proc.*, 38, 2226, 1979.

Berndt, W. O., Renal function tests: what do they mean? A review of renal anatomy, biochemistry, and physiology, *Environ. Health Perspect.*, 15, 55, 1976.

Berndt, W. O., Use of the tissue slice technique for evaluation of renal transport processes, *Environ. Health Perspect.*, 15, 73, 1976.

Cherian, M. G. and Goyer, R. A., Metallothioneins and their role in the metabolism and toxicity of metals, *Life Sci.*, 23, 1, 1978.

Hirsch, G. H., Differential effects of nephrotoxic agents on renal transport and metabolism by use of in vitro techniques, *Environ. Health Perspect.*, 15, 89, 1976.

Hewitt, W. R., Goldstein, R. S., and Hook, J. B., Toxic responses of the kidney, in *Casarett and Doull's Toxicology*, Amdur, M. O., Doull, J., and Klaassen, C. D., Eds., Pergamon Press, New York, 1991, chap. 11.

Roch-Ramel, F. and Peters, G., Micropuncture techniques as a tool in renal pharmacology, *Annu. Rev. Pharmacol. Toxicol.*, 19, 323, 1979.

12

IMMUNOTOXICOLOGY

FUNCTION OF THE IMMUNE SYSTEM

The job of the immune system is to protect the body from harmful invaders. It does this by providing nonspecific barriers to invasion as well as customized defenses against specific threats. The cells which are involved in these processes are commonly known as the white blood cells and include polymorphonuclear leukocytes (PMNs), lymphocytes, and monocytes. These cells originate and mature in the bone marrow and in *lymphatic tissues* including the thymus, spleen, and lymph nodes, and travel throughout the lymphatic and circulatory systems. They communicate with each other and with other cells of the body through the exchange of chemical messengers called *lymphokines*. We will discuss these cells, their functions, and the potential effects of toxicants on the system as a whole.

ANATOMY AND PHYSIOLOGY OF THE IMMUNE SYSTEM

Nonspecific Defense Mechanisms

Nonspecific defense mechanisms create barriers against the entry of invaders in general. For example, the first nonspecific barrier against invasion is the skin. The thickness of the epidermis and the keratin coating help prevent entry of foreign substances into the body, while the secretions of oil and sweat glands (which contain lytic enzymes and antibodies) help wash away and destroy the potential invaders. While the epithelial cells which line the respiratory, gastrointestinal, urinary, and reproductive tracts do not provide as complete a barrier, they do secrete protective mucus and have hairs and cilia which help trap particles.

Some cells of the immune system function as *phagocytes*, engulfing and digesting foreign materials and debris from damaged cells. Examples of phagocytic cells include *macrophages* (which develop from monocytes), and *neutrophils* and *eosinophils*, (two types of PMN cells). Neutrophils and eosinophils are found in the bloodstream, while macrophages are found in tissues (although

they originate as monocytes in the bloodstream). Fixed macrophages are generally immobile, and are found fixed in position in various sites in the body.
Examples include *Kupffer cells* in the liver and *microglia* in the central nervous
system. Free macrophages, on the other hand, can migrate throughout the body.
Macrophages are attracted to the chemicals released by damaged cells, bacteria
and other microbes, and other cells of the immune system.

Another type of cell which is important in nonspecific defense is a type of
lymphocyte known as a *natural killer* (*NK*) cell. Natural killer cells are able to
identify and destroy abnormal cells (cancer cells or cells infected by viruses, for
example). They do this by releasing proteins called *perforins*, which literally
punch holes in the membrane of the target cell, causing its destruction.

There are several groups of proteins found in the bloodstream that contribute
to nonspecific defense. The *complement system* is a set of proteins that work
together to destroy cell membranes, attract phagocytes, and stimulate activity of
various cells of the immune system. Cells which have been infected by viruses
produce proteins called *interferons*, which stimulate uninfected neighboring cells
to produce *antiviral proteins* (*AVPs*). AVPs interfere with viral replication, and
thus slow the spread of the virus. Other proteins called *pyrogens* are released by
macrophages and produce the rise in body temperature that frequently accompanies infections.

If, in spite of the defenses found in skin and blood, an invader manages to
penetrate into underlying tissues, it will encounter one more defense mechanism:
the *inflammatory response* (Figure 1). Damage to tissues stimulates a connective
tissue cell called a *mast cell* to release a number of different chemicals including

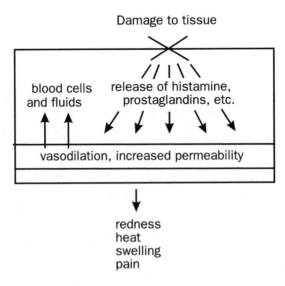

Figure 1   The inflammatory response.

histamine. Histamine produces vasodilation and increased permeability in the blood vessels in the area, bringing increased numbers of macrophages, neutrophils, eosinophils, complement proteins, and other defenders to the area, and aiding in the removal of cellular debris. This increase in blood flow also produces what are often called the "cardinal signs" of inflammation: heat, redness, swelling, and pain. Eventually, fibroblasts are stimulated to lay down collagen, thus producing scar tissue.

Specific Defense Mechanisms

Substances which can activate the body's specific defense mechanisms are called *antigens.* Most antigens are large molecules, and they are usually proteins or at least have a protein component (such as glycoproteins or lipoproteins). Larger structures such as cells or viruses which contain these molecules may also be considered as antigens. To produce a *complete* immune response antigens must be able to both react with *antibodies* (the proteins produced by the specific immune response) and to stimulate the production of more antibodies. To do this, antigens must have at least two sites where antibodies can bind. Molecules which have only one of these *antigenic determinant sites* can react with antibodies, but do not stimulate antibody production. These incomplete antigens, or *haptens*, can stimulate a complete response only by binding to another molecule which can supply the necessary second antigenic determinant site. An example of a hapten is the drug penicillin, which must bind to proteins in the body before producing the well-known allergic response that some individuals display.

The specific immune response itself is carried out by lymphocytes, and consists of two components: a direct attack on the antigen by activated lymphocytes (called *cellular immunity*), and an attack on the antigen by lymphocyte-produced antibodies (called *humoral immunity*).

The type of lymphocytes involved in cellular immunity are called *T cells* (Figure 2). There are many different types of T cells circulating in the bloodstream each of which can be distinguished by the different types of receptors found on their surfaces. These T cells do not respond directly to free antigen, but only to antigens which have been "processed" by other cells. When macrophages or other phagocytic cells engulf antigens, they break them down and then display the fragments on their cell surface. Infected cells also display proteins from the infecting agent on their surfaces. These antigen fragments are bound to cell surface proteins called *HLA* (*human leukocyte antigen*) proteins. HLA proteins are produced by a group of genes called the *MHC* (*major histocompatibility complex*), are found on almost all cells, and serve as unique markers which help the immune system to identify self from nonself. It is this combination of HLA protein and foreign antigen that T cells respond to, with the HLA/antigen combination fitting into the T cell surface receptors in a molecular "lock and key" manner.

When T cells with the proper type of receptor (one with the correct molecular "fit" for that particular antigen) encounter this HLA/antigen combination on a

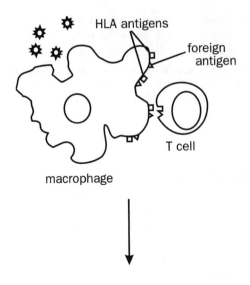

ACTIVATION OF

cytotoxic T cells
helper T cells
supressor T cells
memory T cells

Figure 2
The process of cellular immunity.

cell surface, they bind to the cell and then begin to divide and differentiate into one of several activated forms. *Cytotoxic* (also called "killer") *T cells* attack and destroy antigens directly by secreting cytotoxic chemicals, while *memory T cells* remain dormant, but are poised to react swiftly to any later reappearance of that same antigen. Two other types of T cells are also produced: *helper T cells*, which promote further T cell activation, stimulate phagocytic activity, and assist in the humoral immunity process; and suppressor T cells, which produce a delayed inhibition of both cellular and humoral responses.

Humoral immunity is mediated by lymphocytes called *B cells* (Figure 3). Like T cells, the body has many different types of B cells, which are also differentiated by their surface receptors. Among the proteins found on the surface of B cells are proteins called *antibodies* (sometimes abbreviated Ab) or *immunoglobulins* (sometimes abbreviated Ig) (Figure 4). There are five different classes of antibodies (IgG, IgE, IgD, IgM, and IgA)—each of which plays a different role in humoral immunity. All antibodies consist of a pair of "light" polypeptide chains and a pair of "heavy" polypeptide chains. Both heavy and light chains have a constant region (which does not vary between antibodies of the same class) and a variable region. The variable region is where antibodies recognize and bind antigens.

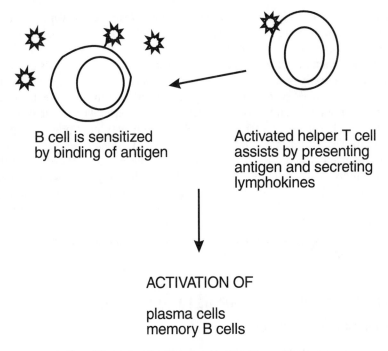

B cell is sensitized
by binding of antigen

Activated helper T cell
assists by presenting
antigen and secreting
lymphokines

ACTIVATION OF

plasma cells
memory B cells

Figure 3   The process of humoral immunity.

When a circulating antigen encounters a B cell with the appropriate antibody
(again, one with the proper molecular shape to bind that antigen) binding occurs,
and the B cell becomes sensitized. For activation to occur, though, the B cell must
also be presented with antigen which is bound to the surface of a helper T cell.

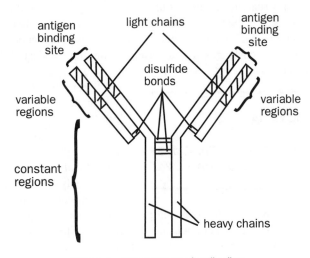

Figure 4   The structure of antibodies.

The activated cell divides and differentiates into *plasma cells*, which produce antibodies, and *memory B cells*, which (like memory T cells) remain dormant unless a later exposure to the same antigen occurs.

Active immunity develops through exposure to the antigen. This exposure may occur naturally or may be deliberate, as in *immunizations*, where individuals are exposed to a dead or inactivated pathogen in order to stimulate the development of immunity and thus avoid getting the disease. This strategy works because of the presence of memory cells, which may continue to respond rapidly for years after the initial exposure. In *passive immunizations*, individuals are injected with antibodies against a particular antigen. These antibodies help the individual's own immune system destroy the antigen. Newborn infants are the beneficiaries of a natural type of passive immunization, as antibodies from the maternal circulation can cross the placenta and enter the fetal circulation. Also, antibodies can be passed to the infant through the mother's breast milk (the infant's digestive tract is "leaky" enough to allow absorption of these large molecules).

EFFECTS OF TOXICANTS ON THE IMMUNE SYSTEM

Toxicant-Induced Allergies

Occasionally, the immune system will respond to an inappropriate stimulus, such as a food component, pollen, dust, or even a drug or toxicant. This response is called a *hypersensitivity response* or *allergic response*. There are four different types of allergic responses. The Type I response is also known as an *anaphylactic* response, and occurs when IgE antibodies are produced, bind to sites on mast cells, and thus produce the release of histamine and other mediators. The results can include skin irritation, rhinitis, asthma, or even rapid systemic vasodilation leading to shock, and usually occur immediately following exposure to an antigen to which the allergic person has become *sensitized*. (Sensitization occurs when a person has been previously exposed and reacted to the antigen and thus has developed memory cells.)

TOLUENE DIISOCYANATE
see also:
   Respiratory toxicology   Ch. 7, p. 98
   TDI   Appendix, p. 247

There are several toxicants which have been observed to produce a Type I response in susceptible individuals. *Toluene diisocyanate (TDI)*, for example, a chemical used in the manufacture of polyurethane, can act as a hapten, combining with body proteins to induce hypersensitivity reactions in exposed individuals. Observations of accidentally exposed workers indicate that the higher the exposure level, the more likely it is that hypersensitivity will develop. Exposure does not necessarily have to be through the respiratory route, as dermal exposure can also produce pulmonary hypersensitivity. These observations have been supported by laboratory studies using the guinea pig, which has proved to be an effective model. Unlike most other allergic reactions, the hypersensitivity induced by TDI may continue after exposure to TDI itself is terminated, perhaps because TDI induces a general increase in reactivity to other irritants.

Another chemical that can elicit a Type I response is the antibiotic *penicillin* (as well as its various derivatives). As with TDI, a metabolite of penicillin acts as a hapten, combining with proteins to provoke the immune response. This response may be mild, or may be quite severe, potentially leading to anaphylactic shock.

Type II responses result when IgG or IgM molecules bind to and destroy blood cells or other cells. Exposure to high levels of *trimetallic anhydrides* (TMAs) can trigger this condition. TMAs may also cause a Type III response, where antigen-antibody complexes become trapped in vascular tissues and produce inflammation.

Type IV responses may take a day or more to develop, and involve the activation and proliferation of T cells. An example of a common type IV response is *allergic contact dermatitis*, also called *sensitization dermatitis*. Individuals may become sensitized to a chemical, often after repeated exposures. One to three weeks after the sensitizing exposure, further exposure to the chemical may lead to the development of an itchy rash, often characterized by the appearance of grouped blisters and edema.

Some of the best-known agents to cause allergic contact dermatitis are the oils contained in the plants *poison ivy* and *poison oak*. These oils act as haptens, combining with proteins in skin to elicit an immune response. When sensitized persons contact the oil, the skin in the area of contact exhibits the sensitization response. (Contrary to public opinion, the fluid which forms in the blisters does not contain the oil itself, and thus contact of this fluid with other parts of the body cannot cause the rash to spread.) The rash generally disappears within 1 to 2 weeks. More serious problems may occur if smoke containing the volatilized oil is inhaled, leading to irritation of the lining of the respiratory tract. Other chemicals which can produce allergic contact dermatitis include *nickel* and *formaldehyde*, as well as some pesticides.

FORMALDEHYDE
see also:
Respiratory toxicology   *Ch. 7, p. 96*
Air pollution   *Ch. 14, p. 206*
Formaldehyde   *Appendix, p. 238*

Toxicant-Induced Autoimmunity

Normally, the immune system learns to distinguish "self" from "nonself" during the process of development. This prevents the immune system from later mounting attacks on normal cells and tissues. When the immune system does inappropriately attack some part of the body, the resulting disease is classified as an *autoimmune disorder*.

Many diseases are now recognized as having a basis in autoimmunity. These include myasthenia gravis (caused by attacks on the neuromuscular junction), multiple sclerosis (caused by attacks on myelin), Type I diabetes (caused by attacks on pancreatic beta cells), and systemic lupus erythematosus (caused by attacks on various body tissues). The possible role of toxicants in triggering these and other autoimmune disorders is now being investigated. Some autoimmune responses may be triggered by exposure to a toxicant with a molecular structure which is similar to the structure of some normal tissue component. In this case, antibodies produced against the toxicant may also react against the normal tissue. Alternatively, toxicants may damage tissue directly exposing in the process tissue constituents which are normally hidden from immune system surveillance. These previously hidden constituents may not then be recognized as "self" by the immune system and thus may be attacked.

Toxicant-Induced Immunosuppression

Immunosuppression, the decreased responsiveness of some or all of the types of cells of the immune system, can be caused by a number of different factors ranging from genetic disorders, to viral infections, to exposure to toxicants. Immunosuppression can even be deliberately induced, as in the case of patients who have undergone organ transplants and hope to avoid rejection of the transplanted tissues, or in the case of patients with autoimmune diseases.

The consequences of immunosuppression depend on the part of the immune system which is affected as well as the degree of suppression. Humoral immunity, cellular immunity, or both may be affected. Consequences which have been observed (both in the laboratory and in epidemiological studies) to accompany immunosuppression include not only increased susceptibility to various types of infection, but also increased risk of cancer (presumably, immune surveillance against abnormal cells is depressed). Also, immunosuppression can diminish the effectiveness of immunizations in preventing future illnesses.

BENZENE
see also:
   Cardiovascular
     toxicology   *Ch. 8, p. 113*
   Benzene   *Appendix, p. 234*

Because of the complexity of the immune system, there are many possible mechanisms by which drugs and toxicants can produce immunosuppression. *Benzene*, for example, is generally cytotoxic to bone marrow, affecting production of white cells, red cells, and platelets. The mechanism of action of benzene is not completely clear, but it does appear that a metabolite of benzene and not benzene itself is responsible for the toxicity. Exposure to benzene has been linked to a decrease in circulating lymphocytes as well as antibodies in humans, and has been shown to lower resistance to infection in rats. *Alkylating agents* (which disrupt DNA replication and thus prevent cell division), *antimetabolites* (which inhibit the synthesis of nucleic acids, again interfering with DNA replication), and radiation exposure also produce general immunosuppression through effects on bone marrow (as well as on other lymphoid tissues where white blood cells are proliferating).

Other immunosuppressants affect the action of lymphokines, the molecules through which the various components of the immune system communicate. The drug *cyclosporine*, for example, inhibits the activation of T cells by inhibiting production of the lymphokine interleukin-2 (IL-2) by helper T cells. *Glucocorticoid hormones* also interfere with lymphokine actions, inhibiting MIF (macrophage migration-inhibitory factor, which keeps macrophages from wandering away), and γ-interferon and interleukin-1 (which stimulate T cells).

Some immunotoxicants act directly on specific lymphoid tissues. Low doses (less than 1 μg/kg) of the compound *2,3,7,8-tetrachlorodibenzo-p-dioxin* (*TCDD*) produces severe damage to the thymus in guinea pigs, with resulting depression in both antibody production and T cell function. While the complete mechanism of action is unclear, the immunosuppressive action of TCDD seems to involve binding to a receptor found in the cytoplasm of thymic epithelial cells. This receptor is also found in hepatocytes, where it is involved in induction of one form of cytochrome P450. Some *organotin* compounds also have direct effects on the thymus.

TCDD	
see also:	
Biotransformation	**Ch. 3, p. 28**
Carcinogenesis	**Ch. 5, p. 59**
Water pollution	**Ch. 15, p. 218**
TCDD	**Appendix, p. 245**

P-450	
see also:	
Biotransformation	**Ch. 3, p. 26**

For many toxicants, though, immune system effects and mechanisms of action are much less well defined. Oral or dermal exposure to *polychlorinated biphenyls* (*PCBs*) lowers circulating antibody levels in mice; however, effects on cellular immunity are not as clear cut. In a number of experiments PCBs suppressed T cell functions, but in other experiments T cell functions were enhanced. In humans,

PCBS AND PBBS	
see also:	
Water pollution	**Ch. 15, p. 219**
PCBs and PBBs	**Appendix, p. 243**

PCB exposure has been associated with decreased antibody levels and increased susceptibility to infection. *Polybrominated biphenyls* (*PBBs*) have also been shown in the laboratory to suppress antibody production, and at higher exposures to suppress cellular immunity as well. In an epidemiological study, a group of Michigan residents who were inadvertently exposed to PBBs through contamination of livestock later displayed a higher percentage of immune system abnormalities than a group of unexposed individuals. However, PCBs and PBBs are known to be contaminated with minute quantities of chlorinated dibenzofurans, compounds with mechanisms of action similar to TCDD, which may be responsible for the observed immunosuppressive effects.

LEAD
see also:
  Reproductive toxicology   Ch. 6, p. 75
  Cardiovascular
    toxicology   Ch. 8, p. 111
  Neurotoxicology   Ch. 9, p. 140, p. 143
  Immunology   Ch.12, p. 180
  Water pollution   Ch. 15, p. 222
  Lead   Appendix, p. 239

Exposure to several metals including *lead* has been shown to have adverse effects on immune function. Lead in drinking water appears to increase susceptibility of rats and mice to bacterial and viral infections, and there is epidemiological evidence that people with elevated blood lead levels (such as workers in the lead industry, or children exposed to lead in paints) may experience the same effects. Lead affects humoral immunity (perhaps through interference with macrophage function) and may or may not affect cellular immunity (the results from different studies have been contradictory). *Cadmium* and *mercury* have similar patterns of activity.

Compounds such as *polycyclic aromatic hydrocarbons* (*PAHs*) and pesticides (including *carbamates*, *organochlorines*, and *organophosphates*) have also been suspected of having immunotoxic effects, and studies on these and other suspected immunotoxicants continue.

METHODS FOR STUDYING IMMUNOTOXICITY

There are several established methods available for studying immune function in the laboratory. The simplest assessments include monitoring white blood cell levels, and looking for changes in weight or abnormal histology in lymphoid tissues. Overall function can be assessed by challenging the immune system of the treated animal by exposing it to bacteria or viruses, and comparing the results (rate of infection or mortality) to results from control animals.

Other tests focus specifically on assessing cellular immunity. These include the mixed lymphocyte response (MLR) assay, which measures the ability of spleen T cells to proliferate when exposed to cells from another individual. The proliferative activity of natural killer (NK) cells can be measured in much the same manner. Other assays have been designed to measure phagocytic activity of macrophages.

Humoral immunity can be assessed through quantification of plasma anti-body levels, perhaps in response to an "antigenic challenge" in the form of an injection of a stimulus such as sheep red blood cells. Another way to quantify antibody production is to count the antibody-producing cells in the spleen following such an antigenic challenge.

REFERENCES

Arndt, K. A., Skin disorders, in *Occupational Health*, Levy, B. S. and Wegman, D. H., Eds., Little, Brown, and Company, Boston, 1983, chap. 19.

Cohen, I. R., The self, the world, and autoimmunity, *Sci. Am.*, April, 1988, 52.

Dean, J. H., Cornacoff, J. B., Rosenthal, G. J., and Luster, M. I., Immune system: evaluation of injury, in *Principles and Methods of Toxicology*, Hayes, A. W., Ed., Raven Press, New York, 1989, chap. 26.

Dean, J. H. and Murray, M. J., Toxic responses of the immune system, in *Casarett and Doull's Toxicology*, Amdur, M. O., Doull, J., and Klaassen, C. D., Eds., Pergamon Press, New York, 1991, chap. 9.

Greenlee, W. F., Molecular mechanisms of immunosuppression induced by 12-*O*-tetradecanoylphorbol-13-acetate and 2,3,7,8-tetrachlorodibenzo-*p*-dioxin, in *Immunotoxicology and Immunopharmacology*, Dean, J. H., Luster, M. I., Munson, A. R., and Gardner, D. E., Eds., Raven Press, New York, 1985, 245–254.

Handschumacher, R. E., Immunosuppressive agents, in *Goodman and Gilman's The Pharmacological Basis for Therapeutics*, Gilman, A. G., Rall, T. W., Nies, A. S., and Taylor, P., Eds., Pergamon Press, New York, 1990, chap. 53.

Lampe, K. F., Toxic effects of plant toxins, in *Casarett and Doull's Toxicology*, Amdur, M. O., Doull, J., and Klaassen, C. D., Eds., Pergamon Press, New York, 1991, chap. 23.

Lawrence, D. A., Immunotoxicity of heavy metals, in *Immunotoxicology and Immunopharmacology*, Dean, J. H., Luster, M. I., Munson, A. R., and Gardner, D. E., Eds., Raven Press, New York, 1985, 341–353.

Nossal, G. J. V., Life, death and the immune system, *Sci. Am.*, 269(3), 52, 1993.

Sharma, R. P. and Reddy, R. V., Toxic effects of chemicals on the immune system, in *Handbook of Toxicology*, Haley, T. J. and Berndt, W. O., Eds., Hemisphere, Washington, 1987, chap. 15.

Thomas, P. T. and Faith, R. E., Adult and perinatal immunotoxicity induced by halogenated aromatic hydrocarbons, in *Immunotoxicology and Immunopharmacology*, Dean, J. H., Luster, M. I., Munson, A. R., and Gardner, D. E., Eds., Raven Press, New York, 1985, 305–313.

13   ECOLOGICAL TOXICOLOGY

INTRODUCTION

A relatively new area within the field of toxicology is *ecological toxicology*, or *ecotoxicology*. Whereas classical toxicology is concerned with assessing effects of toxicants on the molecular, cellular, or physiological levels, ecological toxicology focuses on effects on populations, communities, and ecosystems. This chapter reviews some basic principles of ecology, and discusses effects of toxicants on the population, community, and ecosystem levels and how they can be measured. This chapter focuses more on general principles, with specific environmental toxicants discussed in the chapters on air and water pollution and hazardous waste.

EFFECTS OF TOXICANTS AT THE POPULATION LEVEL

Population Genetics

There are, of course, many different kinds of organisms in the world. Organisms which are structurally and functionally similar and have the ability to produce offspring together are considered to belong to the same *species*. A *population* is a group of organisms of the same species which occupy the same area at the same time.

Some people who study populations focus on *population genetics*, studying changes in the *gene pool* (the sum of all genes in a population). Normally, each individual has two copies of each of their genes (one from each parent). In a population, all copies of a gene may be identical, or there may be two or more variations called *alleles*. For any given gene, then, individuals within the population may have two identical alleles (in which case they are said to be *homozygous* for that gene) or may have two different alleles (in which case they are said to be *heterozygous* for that gene). The assortment of alleles which an individual possesses is their *genotype*, while the physical characteristics they display is their *phenotype*.

In a population, as individuals mate and produce offspring, alleles for each gene are passed onto the next generation in various combinations. It can be mathematically demonstrated that this reshuffling of alleles from generation to generation should not, however, change the overall frequency of a given allele in the gene pool (a principle called the Hardy-Weinberg law; Figure 1). The frequencies of the alleles in a population can then be used to calculate the expected frequency of genotypes, which also should not vary from generation to generation (a state called Hardy-Weinberg equilibrium).

Hardy-Weinberg equilibrium is, in fact, not typically seen in populations because a number of factors tend to disrupt it. Changes in the gene pool, especially in small populations, can be produced by random fluctuations, disasters that dramatically reduce population size, immigration and emigration, and spontaneous mutations.

The most important factor which can alter Hardy-Weinberg equilibrium is *natural selection*. The concept of natural selection is based on observations that in

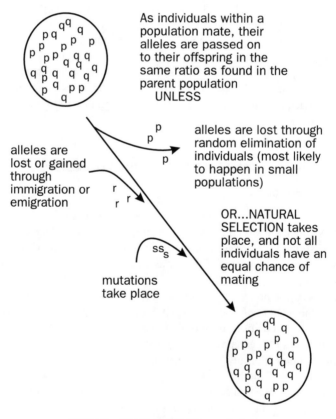

Figure 1   The Hardy-Weinberg principle.

any population: (1) more individuals are born than will live to reproduce, (2) that individuals in a population vary in any number of traits, (3) that variations in traits can be inherited, and (4) that those individuals whose traits give them an advantage in survival and reproduction (in other words, those individuals who are more "fit" for survival) are most likely to survive to pass those traits onto the next generation. Natural selection can alter allele frequencies by favoring a particular genotype which confers some fitness advantage. Individuals with this genotype are more likely to survive to reproduce, and thus pass on their alleles with a greater frequency than individuals of other genotypes. The results of natural selection is that each succeeding generation of a population should become better adapted to its environment.

Characteristics of an environment which influence natural selection are called *selection pressures*. Introduction of toxicants into an environment can exert strong selection pressures favoring or disfavoring particular characteristics. In the classic example, prior to the Industrial Revolution, the light-colored form of the English peppered moth (a moth which frequents tree trunks and rocks) was much more prevalent than the dark-colored form (which presented an easy target for predators against the light background). Once soot began to blacken the trees and rocks, however, the light-colored moth became more conspicuous and within a few years almost all peppered moths were of the dark variety.

Another example of selection pressures exerted by toxicants is the effect of pesticides on target species. Random mutations may render a pest species *resistant* to a particular pesticide. Many cases of resistance occur when a single mutation alters a target protein, making it less sensitive to attack by the pesticide. Recent analysis has shown, however, that some cases of resistance have been due to *amplification* of genes, where many extra copies of a particular gene are found in resistant individuals.

When exposed to a pesticide, the individuals in a population which are most resistant to its effects are those most likely to survive and reproduce. Thus, alleles responsible for pesticide resistance are passed on, and each successive generation becomes more resistant to the pesticide. Development of resistance to a pesticide has been observed in hundreds of species of insects, weeds, fungi, and other organisms. Resistance may develop in response to exposure to pollutants, also. The magnitude of these effects is greatly determined by the genetic makeup of the population and the number of individuals within the population which are exposed.

Development of resistance also occurs in microbes exposed to antibiotics. The use of antibiotics as growth promoters in animal feed has raised concerns that antibiotic-resistant strains of bacteria are being selected for in these animals. These antibiotic-resistant strains may have the potential to infect people, or may pass resistance-carrying alleles to other bacterial species. There has been at least one well-documented case where an antibiotic-resistant strain of *Salmonella* was apparently transmitted to people through infected beef, causing illnesses and deaths.

In the future, it is also likely that the gene pool will be affected more and more by genetic engineering. Recombinant organisms (for bioremediation, for pest resistance in crops, etc.) will be released with greater and greater frequency into the environment. Effects of the introduction of such organisms will be difficult to predict, and careful assessment of the risks and benefits attending their use will be necessary.

Population Growth and Dynamics

Some ecologists study the size and characteristics of populations. Populations grow in size due to natality (births) and immigration and decrease in size due to mortality (deaths) and emigration. The net effect on population size depends on the balance between these opposing factors. If we ignore immigration and emigration, population growth can be modeled very simply by using the equation:

$$\frac{\Delta N}{\Delta T} = rN$$

N = number of individuals in population
T = Time

This equation reflects the fact that population growth is proportional to the number of individuals in the population. The factor r is the *intrinsic rate of increase* of the population, and is a measure of the balance between rates of natality and mortality. Organisms with high r factors are called *r strategists*. They reproduce early and often, with only a small percentage of offspring surviving to adulthood.

Populations do not, however, grow indefinitely. For any population there is a *carrying capacity, K*, which is the maximum number of individuals which can be supported by the environment. As the population nears the carrying capacity, the growth rate slows and eventually the population size stabilizes. Population size for r strategists tends to oscillate relatively rapidly from just above to just below carrying capacity. Other organisms, however, tend to maintain a steady population size just at the carrying capacity (Figure 2). These *K strategists* are characterized by much lower reproductive rates, and longer life spans than r strategists.

Many factors affect carrying capacity, and thus population size. The effects of *density-dependent factors* intensify with increases in population *density* (the number of individuals per some unit area). One example of a density-dependent factor is competition for resources (food, water, shelter, etc.) between members of the same population. The higher the population density, the more intense the competition for finite resources. Another density-dependent factor is predation. The higher the population density of a prey population, the more successful predators are likely to be. (We will discuss predator–prey interactions in more detail in the community section of this chapter.)

Density-independent factors, on the other hand, affect populations in ways which are not dependent on population density. Drastic weather changes, for example, may kill many individuals in a sensitive population.

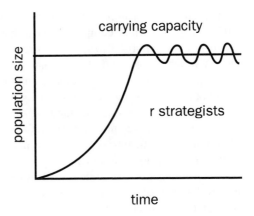

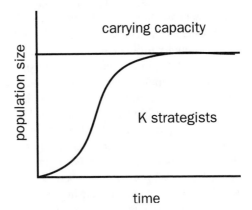

Figure 2
Population size and carrying capacity.

Toxicants, in many cases, may act on populations in a density-independent fashion. For example, a chemical spill into an aquatic environment might be expected to kill a percentage of the individuals in a given population, regardless of whether the population is large or small. Toxicants can also interact with other factors in a density-dependent manner. Toxicants which produce sublethal effects may render individuals more susceptible to infection, for example. This may have a greater effect in crowded populations where pathogens may be more easily transmitted. In general, r strategists can rebound much more quickly from toxicant-induced reductions in population size than can K strategists.

EFFECTS OF TOXICANTS AT THE COMMUNITY LEVEL

All the populations living in the same area at the same time comprise a unit called a *community*. Ecologists who study communities study both community structure as a whole and the interactions between individual species within the community.

One of the most important characteristics of a community is the type and number of species which comprise it. This characteristic is often termed *biodiversity*. It is also important to measure the relative abundance of each species. Species which are particularly abundant, or which play particularly important roles in the structure or function of a community are called *dominant* species. The type of community which develops in a given area depends on factors such as climate, soil, and other physical conditions. A relatively stable community which is characteristic of a given region is called the *climax community* for that region.

Community structure is not always static, but may change over time, particularly in response to environmental change. Changes in the structure and composition of a community over time is called *succession*. Primary succession refers to the development of a community on a previously uncolonized area; secondary succession refers to changes which occur following some perturbation of an existing community. During each of the various stages of succession, organisms dominate which are best able to adapt to the current conditions. These organisms, in turn, affect conditions in such a way as to allow other species to survive and prosper. These changes continue until a stable stage evolves, which is usually the climax community for the region.

Along with physical conditions, the other major factors involved in the determination of community structure are the interactions between different populations within the community. For example, different species may *compete* for a common resource. In fact, two species which are too similar in resource and environmental requirements (in other words, too similar in their *niche*, or role that each plays in the community) generally cannot coexist in the same community. Other interactions include *predation* (where the predator survives by killing and eating the prey), *parasitism* (where the parasite derives nourishment from the host, but generally without causing the host's death), and *mutualism* (where both species gain some advantage from a relationship).

Toxicants can affect community structure and function in several ways. Effects on a particularly sensitive population may not be limited to that population, but may affect other populations with which that species interacts (Figure 3). These interactions are not, however, always easily predictable. Elimination of species through effects of toxicants will in many cases lead to a decrease in biodiversity within a community. Sometimes, however, this is not the case. For example, elimination of a dominant insect competitor through pesticide use may actually increase biodiversity by allowing a more equitable competition for (and thus sharing of) resources by a greater number of species.

Predator–prey interactions can also be affected by the introduction of toxicants into the environment. Reduction in the number of individuals in a prey population, for example, may also adversely affect one or more predators which depend on that particular prey for a substantial portion of their diet. Likewise, loss of a major predator species can also have a significant impact on community structure. Removal of predation pressure can either lead to an increase in biodiversity if more species are allowed to flourish OR a decrease in biodiversity if the

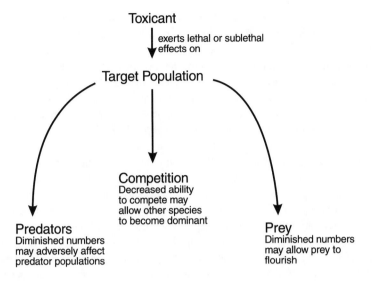

Figure 3   Effects of toxicants on communities.

absence of predation allows one species to become dominant. Sublethal effects of toxicants on predator or prey may also perturb normal predator–prey dynamics.

EFFECTS OF TOXICANTS AT THE ECOSYSTEM LEVEL

A community together with its physical environment comprises an *ecosystem*. There are many different types of terrestrial and aquatic ecosystems, each with their own unique properties which must be considered when studying the effects of pollutants. Two processes which are commonly studied in ecosystems are energy flow and material cycling. Toxicants can disrupt either one of these.

Energy Flow in Ecosystems

The initial source of energy for ecosystem processes comes from the electromagnetic radiation emitted by the sun. *Autotrophs* are organisms with the capability of trapping this electromagnetic energy and storing it in the chemical bonds of molecules such as glucose. These organisms (plants, protists, bacteria) that build energy-storing molecules function as *producers* in the ecosystem.

The rate at which energy is stored by producers is called the *primary productivity* of the ecosystem. Of this energy, some is used by the producers themselves to maintain physiological processes necessary for their own survival. The excess energy remains stored in the molecules which makeup the structure of the organisms, or in other words, in the *biomass* of the organisms.

The second level of organisms in an ecosystem are the organisms which feed directly on the consumers. These organisms are the *primary consumers* or *herbi-*

vores, such as some insects, mammals, and birds. Of the energy these organisms consume, some goes to maintaining their physiological processes, and some is stored in their own biomass. *Secondary consumers* or *carnivores* (such as many amphibians and some mammals), in turn, feed on primary consumers. *Omnivores* may feed on both producers and primary consumers. The energy remaining in organic waste products (including dead organisms) is used by *detritivores* such as bacteria and fungi. Graphic representations of the feeding relationships between different organisms in an ecosystem are called *food webs*.

Each of these levels of organisms (producers, primary consumers, secondary consumers, etc.) is called a trophic level, and the biomass at each trophic level is less than that at the level below. This is because the organisms at each level use some of the energy they receive from the level below, and therefore have less to store as biomass. This concept can be visualized with an energy pyramid, showing the relative amount of stored energy available at each level (Figure 4).

Because of the tight interrelationships between levels, the impact of a toxicant which affects organisms at one level has the potential to spread to other levels as well. For example, toxicant exposure has the potential to decrease productivity in both terrestrial and aquatic ecosystems. This toxicant-induced biomass reduction in producers may then lead to even longer-lasting and more significant biomass reductions at higher trophic levels. This enhanced effect is partly because producers tend to be r strategists while secondary consumers tend to be K strategists. Toxicants which affect detritivores may also impact the entire ecosystem by preventing metabolism and release of nutrients for use by producers. For example, studies have shown that metal-contaminated leaf litter is broken down at a slower rate than non-contaminated litter. Changes in soil pH can also impair detritivore function.

Material Cycling in Ecosystems

The cycling of substances such as water, nitrogen, carbon, and phosphorus through an ecosystem is also critical to ecosystem health. In the *hydrologic cycle*, water molecules cycle between the ocean, ice, surface water, groundwater, and

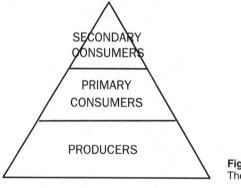

Figure 4
The trophic pyramid.

the atmosphere. In the *nitrogen cycle*, nitrogen in the atmosphere is converted by bacteria to ammonia, nitrite, and nitrate. Plants can absorb ammonia and nitrate, and incorporate them into proteins. Animals then get their necessary nitrogen by consuming plant products. Other soil bacteria convert nitrogen-containing organic wastes back into ammonia. Some bacteria are also capable of converting nitrogen containing organic compounds back into gaseous nitrogen. Other important cycles are the *carbon cycle* and the *phosphorus cycle*. These cycles can be disrupted. The carbon cycle, for example, has been altered by the increased input of carbon dioxide resulting from combustion of fossil fuels (Figure 5). This may ultimately lead to significant changes in global climate.

An understanding of material cycling is important in ecotoxicology because toxicants which are released into ecosystems also cycle. Toxicants may be transported as gases or particulates through the air, dissolved or adsorbed on the surface of particles in the water, or may leach through soils. *Residence times* may be calculated by dividing the total mass of a toxicant by the rate of change (input or output). Residence times for toxicants in the atmosphere are often only a few days, while toxicants in water may have residence times of weeks or months. The residence times for toxicants in soils, however, tend to be much longer: often for hundreds or thousands of years. Sediments on the bottoms of lakes, streams, and oceans may become "sinks" for pollutants, potentially exposing bottom-dwelling organisms to toxicants for many years.

Toxicants in the environment may also be carried by or concentrate in biological tissues through physical processes (such as filter feeding) or through chemical processes. Nonpolar, lipophilic compounds in particular tend to *bioconcentrate*. The bioconcentration factor of a toxicant is the ratio of the concentration

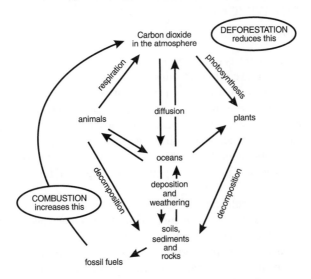

Figure 5   The carbon cycle and potential alterations.

in a particular organism to the concentration of the toxicant in the environment. In general, the higher up in a food web, the more susceptible an organism may be to effects due to bioconcentration.

One example where bioconcentration played an important role is in the actions of the pesticide DDT. Although levels of DDT in small aquatic species was lower than 1 ppm, levels in birds of prey (carnivores at the top of the food web) reached as high as 25 ppm. These levels were sufficient to interfere with eggshell formation, dramatically reducing the numbers of viable offspring in affected populations. Increasing bioconcentration through the food web does not always occur, however. For some metals, bioconcentration is highest in the producers, and declines at higher trophic levels.

BIOTRANSFORMATION
see also:
   Biotransformation   *Ch. 3, p. 21*

Toxicants may move through the environment unchanged, or may be altered through chemical or biological interactions. Some toxicants undergo abiotic transformation, reacting with chemicals in the environment, while others may be metabolized by bacteria or other species. For some compounds these changes may lead to detoxification, but for other relatively nontoxic compounds, the end result may be activation or transformation to a more toxic form. Metals, for example, may be methylated by microorganisms to form more toxic organometals.

EXAMPLES OF ECOSYSTEMS AND VULNERABILITY TO IMPACT BY TOXICANTS

Marine Ecosystems

Water in the *oceans* is in the form of *salt water*, with a salt concentration of 35%. Water temperature can range from very cold for water near the poles and near the ocean bottoms to very warm for surface waters near the equator. Waves and currents move both surface and deep waters. The oceans can be divided into zones (Figure 6). The *littoral* and *neritic* zones are the most productive. The greatest biodiversity is found here, where many different species of *phytoplankton* (photosynthetic protists), *zooplankton* (herbivorous protists), and *nekton* (free-swimming organisms) live. The *benthos*, too, supports a high degree of biodiversity, even in very deep regions.

The open ocean is vulnerable to several different types of pollutants. Some of the most serious problems are accidental oil spillage and leakage, deliberate offshore dumping of hazardous and radioactive wastes, and disposal of nondegradable plastics such as fishing line and nets or plastic soda can rings.

Probably the most significant pollution problems in the ocean, though, occur in the areas where aquatic and terrestrial ecosystems meet—the shore-

OIL SPILLAGE
see also:
Water pollution   *Ch. 15, p. 213*
Petroleum products Appendix, p. 243

lines. *Rocky shores* and *sandy shores*, particularly in popular resort areas, suffer from impacts such as habitat destruction and sewage disposal. The same threats that affect the open ocean (oil, plastic debris, hazardous waste) can also wash up onshore, causing problems. Specialized shoreline ecosystems such as *coral reefs* (tropical offshore structures built from the skeleton of animals called corals) and marine wetlands such as *salt marshes* or *mangrove forests* can also be affected. *Estuaries* (areas, typically at the mouth of a river, where fresh water meets salt water) are particularly vulnerable to pollution. They may receive heavy pollutant loads from upriver, from the ocean, and finally from municipal, agricultural, and industrial activities concentrated around the estuary itself. Because many important commercial fish and shellfish harvesting operations are located in estuaries, pollution of these areas can have significant economic as well as ecological impact.

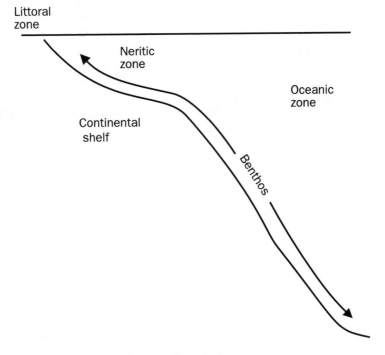

Figure 6   Zones in the ocean.

Freshwater Ecosystems

Lakes and *ponds* are examples of *lentic*, or still water, ecosystems. They are inland depressions filled with water, which may be formed when glaciers gouge out the land or when streams become dammed (either by natural or manmade processes). Lakes, like the oceans, can be divided into zones (Figure 7). As in the ocean, the most productive and diverse zone is the *littoral*. Emergent and floating plants, insects, and fish dominate this zone. The *limnetic* zone contains mostly phytoplankton and zooplankton, along with some fish.

In temperate climates (climates which have changing seasons), lakes go through seasonal changes (Figure 8). The density of water varies with tempera-ture, with the highest density at 4°C. Because of this, in the summer, lakes become *stratified*, with the warmest (lowest density) water at the surface, and pro-gressively cooler, denser water at greater depths (down to 4°C on the floor). Because mixing does not occur, oxygen remains highest at the surface where it enters the water through diffusion or is produced by phytoplankton. Organic material and nutrients, on the other hand, become concentrated near the bottom. Pollutants, also, may not disperse evenly through the lake but may be concen-trated in a particular layer leading to the development of higher concentrations of toxicants than might be otherwise predicted.

In the fall, the water on the surface cools, becomes more dense, and sinks. The next warmest layer is then moved to the surface where it, in turn, cools and sinks. Eventually, the whole lake approaches the same temperature, and waters throughout the lake mix. This is called *overturn*. In the winter, stratification occurs again, except with the coldest waters (0°C) at the surface and progressively warmer, more dense layers below (again, down to 4°C on the bottom). Then, in the spring, as the surface waters warm, overturn occurs again, mixing oxygen, nutrients, and also toxicants throughout the lake.

As lakes age, they tend to become more shallow. Runoff from surrounding areas and silt from streams bring in sediment and organic matter which is deposited

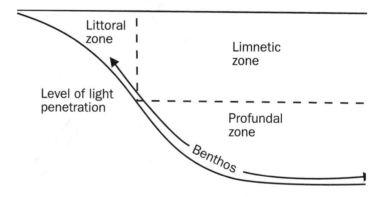

Figure 7   Zones in lakes.

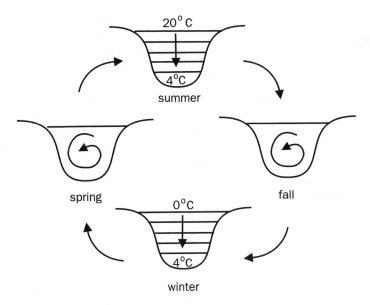

Figure 8 Lake stratification and overturn.

on the bottom of the lake. This input adds nutrients to the ecosystem. Young lakes are usually *oligotrophic*, or nutrient poor. Older lakes are *eutrophic*, or nutrient rich. This input of nutrients generally stimulates plant growth, and

CULTURAL EUTROPHICATION
see also:
Water pollution   *Ch. 6, p. 220*

eutrophic lakes are frequently characterized by a heavy growth of algae. Excessive input of sediments and nutrients as a result of human activities around a lake can lead to accelerated aging of a lake—a phenomenon called *cultural eutrophication.*

The qualities of *lotic* (moving water) ecosystems such as *rivers* and *streams* are determined by several different variables including the characteristics of the channel and the nature of the surrounding terrain, as well as climate conditions such as annual rainfall. Upstream, near the source, rivers and streams tend to be faster moving, eroding sediment from the bottom which will later be deposited downstream as velocity slows. Typically, rivers and streams consist of alternating *riffles*, which are areas of rapid and turbulent flow, and *pools*, which are deeper and have slower flow. Moss and algae grow attached to rocks in the stream bed, and insects and fish live in both fast- and slow-moving areas.

In the processes of material cycling and energy flow, lotic ecosystems receive a good deal of input from outside sources (organic matter falling or being washed into the water, overland runoff, precipitation, or seepage from the ground). Toxicants also enter the ecosystem in this manner. Historically, indus-

RIVER POLLUTION
see also:
    Water pollution   *Ch. 15, p. 211*

trial and municipal waste has been dumped into nearby rivers with little or no treatment. Agricultural runoff containing pesticides and fertilizers has also been a problem.

Freshwater wetlands, too, are impacted by water pollution. Freshwater wetlands can be defined as land areas which are periodically saturated with water. Examples include *marshes* (characterized by grasses as dominant vegetation), *swamps* (wooded wetlands), and *bogs* (wetlands dominated by sphagnum moss). Wetlands serve as important wildlife habitats, and high concentrations of toxicants can threaten the survival of many species. Wetlands are often destroyed to provide land for agricultural or other commercial uses.

Terrestrial Ecosystems

The *tundra* occurs both at high latitudes (*arctic tundra*) and at high altitudes (*alpine tundra*), where the weather is so cold that much of the ground remains frozen all year round. In the summer, the upper layers of the ground may thaw, but the lower levels will remain frozen. Thus, the water released by the thaw remains on the surface, forming wetlands. Because the ground is so cold, activity of the decomposers in the soil is much slower than in warmer climates. Thus, nutrient turnover is limited. Dominant vegetation consists of moss, lichens, and grasses. In the summer, insects are abundant, as are birds (many of which nest in the wetlands) and mammals such as hare, caribou, and wolf.

The tundra is an example of a fragile ecosystem, meaning that it is slow to recover from perturbations. Several of the world's oil fields occur under the tundra, and as a result this ecosystem has been exposed to significant pollution problems. Oil spills and leaks are always a threat. Evidence has shown, however, that tundra vegetation can recover, although slowly, from such spills. Another threat is the additional organic waste produced by human colonization of once remote areas (remember, rate of decomposition is quite slow). The *Arctic National Wildlife Refuge (ANWR)* is an example of a tundra ecosystem that some individuals would like to open up for oil exploration and others would prefer to see remain as wilderness.

The dominant feature of *grasslands* is grass. This ecosystem is also the home to many insects and small, burrowing mammals. Grassland ecosystems are characterized by moderate rainfall which is frequently seasonal in nature. Fire is often an important force in maintenance of grasslands.

Unfortunately, much of the world's original grassland ecosystems have been converted to farming and grazing lands. The tallgrass and shortgrass prairies of North America, the pampas of South America, the veld of Africa, and the steppes of Eurasia have all been severely impacted. As far as effects of toxicants, probably the greatest threat to remaining grasslands is the contamination by pesticides used to manage adjacent agricultural lands.

Deserts are characterized by low rainfall, typically occurring as infrequent heavy cloudbursts. Temperatures in a desert may fluctuate widely during the day, ranging from very warm during the day to very cool at night. Dominant vegetation types are cacti and shrubs, and animals include insects, reptiles, birds, and mammals. Deserts are fragile ecosystems and in many parts of the world are threatened by the pollution which accompanies human activities such as oil drilling. People also frequently attempt to farm and graze on the marginal lands surrounding deserts. Overgrazing or loss of topsoil there can lead to "desertification" of these lands. Improper irrigation can also create problems. Evaporation of irrigation water can leave a residue of salts which are toxic to many desert plants.

There are many different types of *forests*. The *taiga* is a forest found at high altitudes and latitudes that is dominated by coniferous trees. *Temperate forests* occur in temperate zones and may be coniferous, deciduous, or mixed. *Tropical rain forests* occur where rainfall is heavy and even and the temperature is warm year round. These ecosystems are all subjected to destruction through logging and also to air and water pollution caused by industrial activities (including logging, mining, and operation of power plants), and are vulnerable to erosion.

AIR POLLUTION
see also:
  Air pollution   *Ch. 14, p. 201*

ECOTOXICOLOGICAL TESTING METHODS

Single Species Testing

Classic single species toxicology testing, of the type discussed throughout this book, plays an important role in ecological toxicology. The difference is that instead of pursuing a goal of better understanding the effects of toxicants on human health (a direction in which most toxicological research is focused) ecotoxicologists are interested in better understanding the effects of toxicants on a variety of species. As such, it is more appropriate to work with a variety of species, including nonmammalian species such as insects, mollusks, amphibians, fish, or birds. Typical test organisms may include algae, daphnids, shrimp, honey bees, quail, trout, and fathead minnows.

Aquatic toxicity tests are often somewhat difficult to design, due to the complex chemistry of water. Water temperature, pH, ion concentrations, suspended solids, and dissolved gases, among other factors must be closely monitored in order to accurately model real-world conditions. Systems can be either *static*, where water in the system is not changed during the test, or *flow-through*, where water is constantly removed and replenished. Flow-through systems, although more difficult to setup and maintain, are better both for providing acceptable water quality and for maintaining stable toxicant concentrations.

Most ecotoxicological testing to this point has focused less on mechanisms of action of toxicants, and more on identifying endpoints with which to quantify toxicity. Although measurement of the relationship between dose and mortality (the classic LD_{50}) is usable in many situations, a more straightforward and directly applicable correlation in ecological toxicology is the one between environmental concentration and mortality. The LC_{50} measures the concentration of toxicant in the environment (often an aquatic environment) that is necessary to produce mortality in 50% of the test population. LC_{50} tests are typically conducted for exposures ranging from 24 to 96 h in length. Sublethal effects such as changes in behavioral patterns (activity, feeding, reproductive, etc.) and effects on oxygen utilization and respiration can also be measured.

LD_{50}
see also:
   Measuring toxicity   **Ch. 1, p. 4**

Many studies focus on identifying species which are particularly sensitive to the effects of a toxicant. These critical organisms (sometimes called *sentinel species*) would be expected to be among the first components of an ecosystem to be affected by the toxicant. Therefore, monitoring the well being of sentinel species can be used as an early warning system for detecting toxicant effects on ecosystem health. This concept is called *biomonitoring*.

Different developmental stages may also have different sensitivities to toxicants. In *early life stage* toxicity testing, organisms are exposed from fertilization through early juvenile stage, and growth and survival are quantified.

Microcosms

Single species tests are, however, insufficient for ecological toxicology testing. Because of their single species design they are, by definition, unsuitable for measuring community and ecosystem level interactions. These effects may be investigated in the laboratory setting by the use of *microcosms*—artificial ecosystems designed to model real-world processes. Microcosms are generally much less complex than a complete ecosystem, containing only a few selected species in an environment generally limited by size.

Terrestrial microcosms (consisting of soil along with resident microorganisms and invertebrates) are often used to study the fate and transport of pollutants (including microbial metabolism), along with pollutant effects on detritivore function. More complex systems may include plants and even some small vertebrates (typically amphibians such as salamanders or toads). Setting up an aquatic microcosm involves the same complications discussed earlier for single species aquatic testing. Systems may be static or flow-through, and can be used to study fate and transport of toxicants as well as predator—prey interactions and behavior.

Field Studies

Study of an actual toxicant-contaminated ecosystem is probably the best way to study the full set of complex interactions which characterize such a system. Samples of biotic and abiotic components can be taken and analyzed by gas chromatography, HPLC, atomic absorption spectroscopy, etc. for toxicant levels. Population sizes can be estimated and monitored through various ecological sampling methods. However, the actual effects of the toxicant can be difficult to determine without either (1) historical data on the area dating back to before contamination occurred, or (2) a similar, uncontaminated ecosystem to use as a basis for comparison.

Mathematical Modeling

Finally, there are a number of ecotoxicological processes which can be modeled mathematically. For example, the fate and transport of a toxicant in an ecosystem may be predicted by using structure, lipid-water partition coefficient, and other physical or chemical properties in conjunction with ecosystem properties such as soil and water chemistry, population levels, and predator–prey relationships. These models can, however, very quickly become tremendously complex. Often, in order to simplify them, assumptions and estimations are made which may or may not be totally valid. Mathematical models are developed and validated through the use of field studies.

REFERENCES

Barthalmus, G. T., Terrestrial organisms, in *Introduction to Environmental Toxicology*, Guthrie, F. E. and Perry, J. J., Eds., Elsevier, New York, 1980.

Connell, D. W. and Miller, G. J., *Chemistry and Ecotoxicology of Pollution*, John Wiley and Sons, New York, 1984, chaps. 4 and 16.

Freedman, B., *Environmental Ecology*, Academic Press, San Diego, CA, 1989.

Leidy, R. B., Aquatic organisms, in *Introduction to Environmental Toxicology*, Guthrie, F. E. and Perry, J. J., Eds., Elsevier, New York, 1980.

Levin, S. A., Kimball, K. D., McDowell, W. H., and Kimball, S. F., New perspectives in ecotoxicology, *Environ. Manage.*, 8, 375, 1984.

McKim, J. M., Early life stage toxicity tests, in *Fundamentals of Aquatic Toxicology*, Rand, G. M. and Petrocelli, S. R., Eds., Hemisphere, Washington, 1985, chap. 3.

Parrish, P. R., Acute toxicity tests, in *Fundamentals of Aquatic Toxicology*, Rand, G. M. and Petrocelli, S. R., Eds., Hemisphere, Washington, 1985, chap. 2.

Power, E. A. and Chapman, P. M., Assessing sediment quality, in *Sediment Toxicity Assessment*, Burton, G. A., Ed., Lewis, Boca Raton, FL, 1983, chap. 1.

Truhaut, R., Ecotoxicology: objectives, principles, and perspectives, *Ecotoxicol. Environm. Safety*, 1, 151, 1977.

14

AIR POLLUTION

Many of man's activities in our industrialized society produce the unpleasant byproduct of air pollution. This chapter covers the types and sources of air pollution and the potential effects of air pollution on human health and ecosystem function.

TYPES AND SOURCES OF AIR POLLUTANTS

Since the route of exposure for most air pollutants is respiratory, they tend to be categorized in the same manner as other inhaled toxicants: as either *gases* or *particles*. *Primary pollutants* enter the atmosphere directly as a result of some natural or manmade activity or process; *secondary pollutants* are formed when primary pollutants and other atmospheric constituents undergo chemical reactions in the atmosphere.

The major gaseous air pollutants include *carbon oxides* (carbon monoxide and carbon dioxide), *sulfur oxides*, *nitrogen oxides*, *ozone*, and volatile *hydrocarbons* (benzene, methane, and a special class of halogenated molecules called CFCs). Major particulates include *dusts, pollen*, and *heavy metals*. Most of these are produced during the process of *combustion*, the burning of organic matter. In *more developed countries* (*MDCs*), fossil fuels such as oil, gas, and coal are burned for energy and heat, while in *less developed countries* (*LDCs*) wood and other crop matter is burned. The clearing of forests and grasslands by burning also releases pollutants into the atmosphere.

GENERAL EFFECTS OF AIR POLLUTANTS

Exposure to air pollution has been related to increased risk for a number of different adverse effects. Analyzing human health or ecosystem level effects of pollutants is difficult, though, due to the large number of different pollutants and the potential for interactions between them. Effects of two irritant pollutants, for example, are frequently additive. Also, some pollutants may affect the mucociliary escalator, macrophage activity, or one of the other defense mechanisms of the respiratory tract, and thus exacerbate the effects of others.

Levels of pollutants high enough to produce immediate adverse effects on human health frequently occur during a weather condition called a *thermal inversion*. Thermal inversions occur when a layer of warmer air traps a layer of colder air near the surface. This also traps airborne emissions, leading to the development of very high concentrations of pollutants (particularly if the inversion lasts for several days). The most serious inversion-related air pollution episode in this country occurred in Donora, PA in 1948, and led to the death of over 20 individuals. Most of these deaths were due to exacerbation of preexisting respiratory diseases (bronchitis, emphysema, or asthma, for example).

In point of fact, long-term exposure to lower levels of pollutants has been implicated in the development of these same chronic respiratory diseases. Epidemiological evidence points to higher rates of chronic respiratory problems in areas with high levels of pollution. Some cases of lung cancer, too, may be attributable to exposure to air pollutants. Again, firm conclusions are hard to draw, due to confounding factors such as smoking.

Most studies of the effect of air pollutants on ecosystems has focused on effects of pollutants on plant growth and survival. On a molecular level, pollutants interact with plants in much the same way as with humans, producing cellular dysfunction and eventual physiological impairment. In plants, injury to tissues typically occurs in leaves and needles. Injury to plants, which of course as producers function as the base of the trophic pyramid, can have repercussions throughout an ecosystem.

SPECIFIC POLLUTANTS

Carbon Oxides

Carbon monoxide and carbon dioxide make up the carbon oxides. The most significant health effects of *carbon monoxide (CO)* are produced as a result of the high affinity binding of carbon monoxide to the oxygen-carrying molecule hemoglobin. When 2% of circulating hemoglobin is converted to carboxyhemoglobin (the form which is unable to carry oxygen), neurological impairment can be measured. At 5% conversion, cardiac output increases, and other cardiovascular changes are noted. CO also binds to another heme-containing molecule: cytochrome P450.

CARBON MONOXIDE
see also:
   Cellular sites of action   *Ch. 4, p. 49*
   Cardiovascular
      system   *Ch. 8, pp. 110, 114*
   Carbon monoxide   *Appendix, p. 236*

Levels of CO in the atmosphere vary by location, time of day, and time of year, and range from only a few ppm in nonindustrialized areas to 40 or 50 ppm or higher in urban areas. Levels are particularly high inside automobiles and in tunnels and garages. Exposure to environmental levels of 30 ppm CO over 8 h results in the conversion of 5% of circulating hemoglobin.

Increasing levels of *carbon dioxide* (CO_2) in the atmosphere leads to a different set of problems. Carbon dioxide is one of the gases known as *greenhouse gases* which are capable of absorbing the infrared radiation emitted by the earth. Thus, instead of escaping into space this radiation heats the lower levels of the atmosphere, in what has been called the *greenhouse effect* (Figure 1). To some extent, the greenhouse effect is necessary to support life, because without it the temperatures near the earth's surface would very likely be too cold for life to exist. The burning of fossil fuels, however, is releasing CO_2 to the atmosphere at a much higher rate than ever before, and at the same time deforestation is reducing the number of plants able to remove CO_2 from the atmosphere through photosynthesis. The result has been a 20% increase in atmospheric CO_2 over the last 100 years.

Most scientists predict that the increase in levels of CO_2 and other greenhouse gases will lead to an increase in surface temperatures (this predicted increase has been termed *global warming*). One unanswered question is: how high will temperatures go? Some mathematical climatological models have indi-

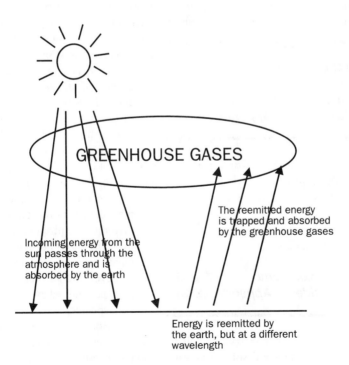

Figure 1 The greenhouse effect.

204 PRINCIPLES OF TOXICOLOGY

cated that average temperatures could rise as much as 5°C overall, with greatest increases at the poles. Other models predict less warming due to offsetting factors such as increased reflection of incoming solar energy by pollutants in the atmosphere. Data collected over the past 100 years indicate a slight increase in average temperatures in many parts of the world, but small changes are difficult to detect as they are easily obscured by the day-to-day variability inherent in climate.

Another set of unanswered questions deals with the effects of global warming on plant and animal life and human survival. Melting of polar ice would lead to rising of the oceans (perhaps by as much as several feet), potentially putting many coastal areas below sea level. Changes in rainfall patterns are also likely which could adversely affect agricultural areas. Shifts in forest composition would be seen, as cold-adapted species die out in southern regions and spread into northern regions. Populations of animals, too, may migrate, moving either to more northern regions, or to higher altitudes. The rapidity of the potential change is a cause for concern for many biologists, however, who wonder if species will have the time to make these adaptations in range and habitat. Many fear that biological diversity will be significantly diminished worldwide.

Sulfur Oxides and Nitrogen Oxides

Both sulfur oxides and nitrogen oxides are pulmonary irritants which are released during the burning of coal and petroleum products. Increases in airway resistance (due to irritation of upper airways) in humans can be seen at exposure levels as low as 5 ppm of *sulfur dioxide* (SO_2). Individuals with asthma or other chronic respiratory conditions may, however, be much more sensitive to the irritant, displaying increases in airway resistance at exposure levels of only 0.5 to 1.0 ppm SO_2.

SULFUR DIOXIDE
see also:
 Respiratory toxicology   Ch. 7, p. 96
 Sulfur dioxide   Appendix, p. 245

Nitrogen dioxide (NO_2), on the other hand, is an irritant which affects the lower airways primarily. There is also some evidence that exposure to NO_2 may cause increased susceptibility to respiratory infection. Concentrations necessary to produce pulmonary effects are, however, higher than are generally encountered even in polluted atmospheres.

NITROGEN DIOXIDE
see also:
 Respiratory toxicology   Ch. 7, p. 97
 Nitrogen dioxide   Appendix, p. 240

Both sulfur and nitrogen oxides can react with hydroxyl radicals in the atmosphere to produce *sulfuric* and *nitric acids* which then dissolve into water droplets. These acids are not only pulmonary irritants, but are the major components of the phenomenon called *acid rain*. Although rain is by nature somewhat acidic, high levels of sulfuric and nitric acids in the atmosphere can produce rain with a pH of 5.5 or lower (rain with a pH as low as 2.6 has been measured!). Acid rain typically does not fall near the source of the sulfur and nitrogen oxides which produce it, but instead the pollutants may travel hundreds of miles (during which time the acids are produced) to fall on areas far downwind.

Acid rain has the potential to affect the structure and function of aquatic ecosystems. Whether or not a lake is affected depends on its surroundings. Lakes in areas rich in limestone and other water soluble alkaline rocks contain bicarbonate and other ions which can neutralize the acid precipitation. Also, if the lake's substrate contains metals such as calcium or magnesium, cation exchange can occur. This process decreases the water's hydrogen ion concentration (and thus raises the pH), but at the same time increases the concentration of heavy metals.

Lakes which lack these natural buffering systems, however, may undergo changes in pH. This acidification in turn affects the many non acid-tolerant species and causes a shift in community composition, potentially reducing biodiversity of fish, zooplankton, and phytoplankton. Lakes in the Adirondack region of New York, for example, have been particularly hard hit by a combination of high levels of acid precipitation (produced by electric/utilities and industry in the upper Midwest) and a lack of natural buffers. Fortunately, studies have indicated that reducing acid input will allow lakes to recover, although return to the initial pH may take many years.

Acid rain can affect terrestrial ecosystems, too. In recent years, forests in Europe and the U.S. have been undergoing a decline that has been attributed at least in part to effects of acid rain. A wide variety of species of trees are affected, in many different locations. Particularly hard hit, however, are the coniferous forests found at high elevations. The mechanism of this effect is not clear, but several hypotheses have been advanced. Through the process of cation exchange, acid rain may leach calcium and magnesium (which are necessary for tree growth) from the soil or from needles and leaves. Also, soil pH may become lowered to the point that soil bacteria and other decomposers are unable to breakdown decaying organic matter and release the nutrients for uptake by trees and other vegetation. These stresses may then combine with other environmental stresses (including other types of air pollutants) to make the trees more susceptible to disease or injury. Lichens and moss are also susceptible to damage from acid rain.

Hydrocarbons and the Formation of Secondary Pollutants (Including Ozone)

Incomplete combustion of fossil fuels and other organic materials leads to the release of hydrocarbons into the atmosphere. There are also some natural sources of atmospheric hydrocarbons, including release of terpenes by plants and the release of methane by decomposers. Hydrocarbons react in the presence of sunlight with oxygen or nitrogen oxides to produce a number of secondary pollutants in the atmosphere. These secondary pollutants include *ozone, aldehydes*, and *peroxyacetylnitrate (PAN)*, a mixture commonly referred to as *photochemical smog*.

OZONE
see also:
  Respiratory
    toxicology   *Ch. 7, p. 97*
  Ozone   *Appendix, p. 242*

Although ozone is a necessary component of the stratosphere or upper atmosphere, it is a pollutant in the troposphere or lower atmosphere. Ozone is a respiratory irritant which affects the lower airways, producing inflammation directly and also causing an increase in reactivity to other irritants (such as other air pollutants and some allergens). Short-term exposure (a few hours) to ozone concentrations on the order of 0.10 ppm has been shown to produce temporary decreases in measured lung volumes in humans. Ozone also affects plants, probably reacting with unsaturated lipids in cell membranes to damage leaves and needles and ultimately to reduce growth. Effects of ozone and PAN on membranes are similar.

FORMALDEHYDE
see also:
  Respiratory toxicology   *Ch. 7, p. 96*
  Immunotoxicology   *Ch. 12, p. 177*
  Formaldehyde   *Appendix, p. 238*

Formaldehyde is a water-soluble irritant which affects the upper respiratory tract. Exposure to as little as 0.3 ppm formaldehyde has been shown to alter respiratory rate. Some laboratory studies have linked exposure to formaldehyde with an increased risk of nasal cancer in rats. Epidemiological studies, however, have not as yet found a strong association between exposure and cancer risk in humans.

Chlorofluorocarbons (CFCs)

Chlorofluorocarbons (CFCs) are a group of stable compounds with several different uses in commercial and industrial processes including use as propellants in aerosol cans, as refrigerants, and in the making of styrofoam and other polystyrene products. Due to their chemical stability, CFCs do not react with other molecules in the lower atmosphere (the troposphere); instead, they travel to the

CHLOROFLUOROCARBONS
see also:
  CFCs   *Appendix, p. 236*

upper atmosphere (the stratosphere) where they catalyze the breakdown of ozone (Figure 2). As a catalyst, the chlorine in CFCs participates in the reaction but yet remains unchanged.

Oxygen molecules are dissociated by ultraviolet light

$$O_2 \xrightarrow{h\nu} O + O$$

An oxygen atom combines with an oxygen molecule to make ozone

$$O + O_2 \longrightarrow O_3$$

A chlorine atom is released from a CFC by ultraviolet light

$$CFC \xrightarrow{h\nu} CFC + Cl$$

A chlorine atom combines with ozone to form chlorine monoxide and an oxygen molecule

$$Cl + O_3 \longrightarrow ClO + O_2$$

Chlorine monoxide reacts with an oxygen atom to regenerate a chlorine atom

$$ClO + O \longrightarrow Cl + O_2$$

Figure 2   Chemical reactions involved in the breakdown of ozone in the atmosphere.

Thus, one CFC molecule may ultimately catalyze the breakdown of tens of thousands of ozone molecules.

The ozone layer in the stratosphere absorbs ultraviolet radiation, protecting life on earth from its adverse effects. Exposure to ultraviolet radiation can increase the risk of skin cancer and cataracts, and can slow plant growth. Scientists have recently measured large holes in the ozone layer over Antarctica, and reductions in thickness of the layer in other parts of the world (including over North America).

Particulates

Particles found in the atmosphere can be divided into two classes on the basis of size and chemical composition. Small particles (<1 μm in diameter) are produced primarily by combustion processes. These particles contain high levels of sulfate and carbon, and tend to be acidic. Larger particles come from mechanical processes, such as weathering

PARTICULATES
see also:
   Respiratory toxicology   *Ch. 7, p. 96*

of rock and soil and are not acidic. Particulates act as irritants, and many of the smaller particulates may contain carcinogenic components.

"Air Toxics"

Other air pollutants which do not fall into the above categories are sometimes referred to as "*air toxics*." One main group of air toxics are the heavy metals such as *mercury*, *lead*, and *cadmium* which are emitted from smelting and other industrial operations. Other air toxics include various *pesticides* and *solvents*.

INDOOR AIR POLLUTION

A growing problem is that of indoor air pollution. As energy conservation measures have led to the construction of "tighter" homes and offices with lower air exchange rates, pollutants that once would have been vented regularly to the outside are now trapped inside for longer periods of time. Cigarette smoke, formaldehyde, and solvents such as trichloroethylene and benzene have all been postulated to be health threats. Most recently, attention has focused on *radon*, a radioactive gas released by the decay of radium and uranium. Radon gas escapes to the surface from the underground rocks and soils in which it is formed—an event that only poses problems if it is then confined by a structure such as a house. In areas where radon release is high, concentrations of radon in homes may reach unacceptable levels (particularly in basement areas). Currently, the EPA defines acceptable levels as below 4 picocuries of radiation per liter of air. There is, however, some discussion among scientists regarding whether or not the significance of health risks from radon exposure may have been somewhat overestimated.

CONTROL OF AIR POLLUTION

The main piece of legislation that regulates levels of air pollutants is the *Clean Air Act*, most recently reauthorized in 1990. The Clean Air Act divided the U.S. into *air quality control regions*, and then set *emission standards* to regulate the amount of pollutants that an industry can release, and *ambient air standards* to specify maximum allowable levels of pollutants in each region. The recent reauthorization set new timetables for meeting these air quality goals, and setup, in addition, an *emissions trading policy*. This policy allows companies to buy and sell permits which allow them to emit sulfur dioxide. Thus, the biggest polluters would have to buy extra permits at market value, while companies which pollute less could sell their additional permits for a profit. Limits on this trading are necessary, though. Additional emissions could not be purchased for use within an air quality region if it meant that ambient air standards would be exceeded.

Industries use many methods to control emissions of air pollutants. Some of these methods are illustrated in Figure 3.

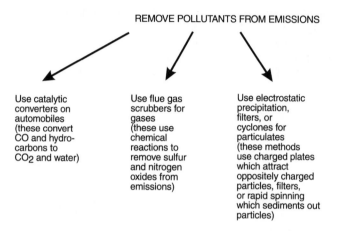

Figure 3   Methods for reducing emissions of air pollutants.

ACCIDENTS RESULTING IN AIR POLLUTION

There have been several major releases of highly toxic compounds into the atmosphere in recent decades. The most notorious examples include the emission of TCDD from a hexachlorophene manufacturing plant in Seveso, Italy, on July 10, 1976. Remediation of the area involved removal of topsoil and there has been a long-term epidemiological study of the population. The respiratory irritant, methyl isocyanate, was released from an underground storage tank in a facility manufacturing carbamate pesticides from this precursor. This accident in Bhopal, India, on Dec. 3, 1984 resulted in many fatalities. A large explosion in a nuclear power plant in Chernobyl, Ukraine, on April 26, 1986 led to severe contamination of the local area with radionuclides as well as radioactive fallout from the airborne plume in parts of eastern Europe and Scandanavia. Rainfall through the atmospheric plume increased the fallout of cesium and the plume was detected around the world in about two weeks.

REFERENCES

Amdur, M. O., Air pollutants, in *Casarett and Doull's Toxicology*, Amdur, M. O., Doull, J., and Klaassen, C. D., Eds., Pergamon Press, New York, 1991, chap. 25.

Cohn, J. P., Gauging the biological impacts of the greenhouse effect, *Bioscience*, 39, 142, 1989.

Heck, W. W. and Anderson, C. E., Effects of air pollutants on plants, in *Introduction to Environmental Toxicology*, Guthrie, F. E. and Perry, J. J., Eds., Elsevier, New York, 1980, chap. 10.

Houghton, R. A. and Woodwell, G. M., Global climatic change, *Sci. Am.*, 260, 36, 1989.

Jones, P. D. and Wigley, T. M. L., Global warming trends, *Sci. Am.*, 263, 84, 1990.

Mohnen, V. A., The challenge of acid rain, *Sci. Am.*, 259, 30, 1988.

Schindler, D. W., Effects of acid rain on freshwater ecosystems, *Science*, 239, 149, 1988.

Schneider, S. H., The changing climate, *Sci. Am.*, Sept., 70, 1989.

Shaw, R. W., Air pollution by particles, *Sci. Am.*, 257, 96, 1987.

White, R. M., The great climate debate, *Sci. Am.*, 263, 36, 1990.

15

WATER POLLUTION

WATER IN THE ENVIRONMENT

Oceans, Lakes, and Rivers

Most (over 97%) of the world's water is in the oceans. The remaining water is found in ice and glaciers, in the ground, in the atmosphere, in lakes and rivers, and in living organisms. The structure and function of the aquatic ecosystems found in oceans, lakes, and rivers have been discussed in Chapter 13.

WATER IN THE ENVIRONMENT
see also:
   Ecotoxicology   *Ch. 15, p. 192*

Groundwater

Water pollution affects not only the aquatic ecosystems which are exposed to it, but can also have an impact on human health. The pollution of groundwater is a special case for concern. Groundwater is found below the surface of the earth, contained in a porous rock structure called an aquifer. Groundwater is a major source of irrigation and drinking water. Aquifers are recharged by surface water which percolates down through the soil, and if the water passes through contaminated areas (hazardous waste disposal sites, near leaking underground tanks, etc.) toxicants may leach out and be carried into the aquifer. Water in the aquifer flows, as does surface water, from higher to lower elevations, but at a rate as slow as a few inches a day. With little mixing and diluting, and few bacteria to decompose waste, toxicant levels may become quite high.

Polluted groundwater may contaminate the lakes and streams which it feeds into, and can lead to human health problems if used for drinking water. The EPA has estimated that almost half of the public water supply systems which rely on groundwater as a source are contaminated with one or more potentially hazardous toxicants.

Almost everywhere water is found, it is vulnerable to pollution. Water pollution is a complex topic—there are many sources and types of water pollutants. Also, water pollutants may react together or with water itself, resulting in altered chemical forms. Because of this, the toxicity of pollutants in the aquatic environment varies with a number of factors (e.g., water temperature, hardness, and pH), and may in fact be very difficult to predict. Protecting our water resources is, however, critical to both ecological and human health.

TYPES AND SOURCES OF WATER POLLUTANTS

Water pollutants are generally classified as belonging to one of several broad groups. Organic substances include dead and decaying plant and animal matter and wastes as well as organic compounds such as petroleum products, solvents, pesticides, and polymers. Inorganic substances include metals, nitrates, and phosphates. *Biological agents* include viruses, bacteria, protozoans, and other parasites which can cause disease. *Suspended matter* includes large, insoluble particles of soil and rock. Finally, *radioactive materials* and *heat* each constitute their own group.

Water pollutants can come from *industrial*, *municipal*, or *agricultural* sources. Industrial sources tend to be of the type called *point sources*, meaning that the emission of pollutants occurs at one or more very specific locations (a discharge pipe, for example). Some municipal sources, such as discharges from sewage treatment plants, are also point sources. Most agricultural sources, on the other hand, are *nonpoint sources*. This means that the emission of pollutants occurs over a wide area, not just at a single point. One example of nonpoint source pollution is the runoff of fertilizer and pesticide-contaminated water from croplands. Urban storm drains are another example. Storm runoff can carry rain-borne pollutants which are less likely to be bound to soil particles than are agricultural chemicals, and thus may pose an even greater threat. Most water pollution is of the nonpoint source variety. Unfortunately, this is the most difficult type to control.

ORGANIC POLLUTANTS

Organic Wastes

As discussed in the chapter on ecological toxicology, energy flows and materials cycle through aquatic ecosystems. Aquatic ecosystems contain producers, consumers, and of course decomposers. Decomposers are the bacteria and other organisms that breakdown dead and decaying organic matter. In the process they obtain energy and release nutrients for reuse by other organisms. Some of these bacteria, particularly those that dwell in the sediments, are *anaerobic*, which means that they perform their metabolic processes without needing oxygen. Typically, the energy repackaging pathways for these bacteria involve either *fer-*

mentation (the conversion of sugar to either lactic acid or ethanol) or a variation of oxidative phosphorylation in which sulfates or nitrates substitute for oxygen as an electron acceptor. Other bacteria, however, are *aerobic*, which means that they require oxygen for their metabolic activities.

Normally, this system is balanced, with the bacterial population size limited by the supply of waste from which they obtain energy. If, however, additional organic waste material is added to the ecosystem (through influx of sewage, or organic waste-containing sediments) the bacterial population may undergo rapid growth. The respiratory activities of all these bacteria can then lead to oxygen depletion, particularly in lakes (the greater surface area of streams combined with the motion of the water help keep the stream oxygen levels high). If oxygen levels drop lower than around 5 mg/l, the survival of species with high oxygen needs may be threatened.

Respiratory activities of the decomposers can be assessed through a measurement called *biological oxygen demand*, or *BOD*. A high BOD indicates that there is a high level of decomposer activity as a result of high levels of organic waste (animal wastes, fertilizer, etc.) in the water.

Petroleum Products

Several million tons of petroleum are spilled or leaked into the oceans every year. Part of this petroleum comes from land-based sources such as municipal and industrial wastes which are dumped into rivers and streams and ultimately find their way into the ocean. The remainder comes from tankers (both accidental spills and routine releases), and leakage from off-shore drilling sites. The most significant recent tanker accidents include the wreck of the *Torrey Canyon* off the southern coast of England in 1967, the grounding of the *Amoco Cadiz* which dumped 230,000 metric tons (MT) of oil into the English Channel in 1978, and the *Exxon Valdez* accident in 1989. One of the biggest single accidents was the IXTOC I drilling rig accident in 1979 which was responsible for the release of 400,000 MT into the Gulf of Mexico. But the biggest oil disaster was the spill which occurred in 1991 during the Persian Gulf war, when an estimated 250 million gallons escaped (twice the volume that was released in the IXTOC accident, and 20 times the volume released by the *Exxon Valdez*).

Petroleum is a complex substance consisting of hundreds of different compounds. The bulk of crude petroleum (also called *crude oil*) is made up of *aliphatic* (straight-chain) *hydrocarbons* with backbones of anywhere

PETROLEUM
see also:
Petroleum products Appendix, p. 243

from 1 to 20 or more carbons. The aliphatic hydrocarbons include compounds such as natural gas (1 to 2 carbons), bottled gas (3 to 4 carbons), gasoline (5 to 10 carbons), kerosene (12 to 15 carbons), fuel and diesel oil (15 or more carbons), and lubricating oils (19 or more carbons). Crude oil also contains *cyclic hydrocarbons*, *aromatic hydrocarbons* (with structures based on benzene), sulfur, nitrogen, and a variety of trace metals.

When oil is spilled or leaks into a waterway, it initially spreads across the surface (forming an *oil slick*). Some of the more volatile components may then evaporate, and because the rate of evaporation depends directly on temperature and surface area, the process is more rapid in warm areas and in rougher seas (which promote formation of droplets of spray). Other components (particularly the aromatics) may dissolve into the water. The remaining heavier material forms an emulsion sometimes called *mousse*, or may eventually form lumps called *tar balls*. Some of the oil is eventually broken down by microorganisms or by photochemical processes.

As with other compounds, toxicity of crude oil components in general correlates well with lipid solubility, because lipid soluble compounds are (1) better able to cross membrane barriers and enter organisms, (2) more likely to be widely distributed in the body (including into the brain) and (3) more likely to be retained in depot fat tissues over time and to bioconcentrate through the food web. Studies of oil spills along rocky shores (the *Torrey Canyon*, *Amoco Cadiz*, and *Exxon Valdez*) have indicated that following release of oil, immediate effects are seen on community structure, with species of green algae replacing the more sensitive red and brown algae. Many populations of invertebrates (including crustaceans, mollusks, and starfish) may be completely destroyed. Some fish populations may also be impacted.

Probably the most dramatic and immediate effects of oil spills, though, are on the birds and mammals. The feathers of seabirds become coated with oil, causing them to lose their capacity to insulate the animal, and resulting in death from hypothermia. In addition, oiling of feathers causes loss of buoyancy, potentially resulting in drowning. Ingestion and systemic toxicity may also occur during attempts by the bird to clean the feathers. Marine mammals such as otters and seals may suffer the same fates, due to similar effects of the oil on their fur. Although estimates are difficult to make, the *Exxon Valdez* spill killed probably close to half a million birds and several thousand marine mammals.

Ironically, analysis of aftermath of the *Exxon Valdez* and other spills has indicated that attempts to clean fouled shores may not, in fact, be ecologically beneficial. Some studies have indicated that recovery is quicker on beaches which have not been cleaned than on beaches that have. For example, scientists have pointed out that cleaning with detergents may do more harm than good, as the detergent/oil mix may produce greater mortality than the oil alone. Also, the use of dispersants to dilute the spill may result in spreading the damage to offshore areas that otherwise might have remained unaffected. Finally, using hot water to blast beaches may not only drive oil deeper into the sediments, but may also kill invertebrates. Thus, there is considerable debate about whether the 2 1/2 billion dollars spent by Exxon on cleanup was particularly effective.

One promising group of experimental techniques for cleaning up spills is grouped together under the term *bioremediation*. One form of bioremediation consists of adding nutrients to the water, thereby ensuring that the natural oil-metabolizing microorganisms have sufficient quantities of these nutrients. This allows the population to grow more rapidly, and hopefully to metabolize more of the oil. Initial studies of the effectiveness of this technique in Prince William Sound, however, were inconclusive. Another bioremediation option is the addition of nonnative oil-metabolizing (perhaps even genetically engineered) microorganisms. Probably the best solution, however, to the oil spill problem is to prevent the spill through use of double-hulled ships (which could contain their oil cargo even if the outer hull is damaged) and better training of crews.

Although many of the most visible effects of an oil spill may disappear after a few months or years, the impact lingers on, particularly in relatively isolated, protected shoreline ecosystems. Because degradation is slow and incomplete, crude oil components find their way into the food chain, and may bioaccumulate to toxic levels. Shellfish, for example, from polluted areas may be unsuitable for consumption. Evidence has shown that traces of oil can be found in sediments and biological tissues for as long as 20 years after the initial spill.

Also, most oil pollution occurs in regions that suffer from chronic exposure to low levels of crude oil (areas near refineries, for example). Again, effects from this type of exposure may not be as dramatic as that resulting from a single incident, but over the long term bioaccumulation and resulting systemic toxicity can affect community and ecosystem structure as well as posing potential health hazards for humans who harvest fish and shellfish from the area.

Pesticides

Pesticides are widely used in our society. They play a role in blocking transmission of vector-borne diseases such as malaria, for controlling insects and weeds in farming, and in maintaining relatively pest-free homes and yards. Because of their widespread use, however, they frequently find their way into aquatic ecosystems. In many cases, pesticides enter waterways as a component of nonpoint source runoff from agricultural lands. Aerial application of pesticides can also result in water pollution, as pesticide may drift downwind and be deposited in lakes or rivers. Pesticides may even be deliberately introduced, in order to limit growth of algae or control insects.

Both routine industrial effluent emissions and accidental spills from pesticide manufacturing facilities can also contaminate aquatic ecosystems, as can urban runoff. In 1986, for example, a fire at the Sandoz warehouse near Basel, Switzerland led to the release of more than one thousand tons of pesticides into the already polluted Rhine River. Pesticides may also leach out of hazardous waste disposal facilities and enter groundwater.

The behavior of pesticides in an aquatic ecosystem depends mainly on the chemistry of the pesticide itself. Pesticides vary widely, for example, in lipid solubility as well as *persistence* in the environment (a measure of the amount of time the pesticide remains in the environment before being broken down). Pesticides may dissolve in the water, may adsorb to the surface of particles in the water, or may be absorbed by aquatic organisms. Of course, the more lipid soluble the pesticide, the more likely it is to be absorbed by an organism, partition into fat tissues, and be passed along through the food chain in the process of bioconcentration. Many pesticides undergo both metabolism by bacteria and other organisms and other nonenzymatic photochemical alterations.

One major category of pesticides is *chlorinated hydrocarbon insecticides*. Pesticides in this group include the dichlorodiphenylethanes, the cyclodienes, and the hexachlorocyclohexanes (Table 1). *DDT*, a dichlorodiphenylethane, is a persistent insecticide. This biologically active compound is initially metabolized to breakdown products which are also biologically active, and which are only slowly converted to inactive forms. The half-life of DDT in the environment is generally estimated at between 2 and 3 years. Because of its low water solubility and high lipid solubility, DDT does not dilute out in aquatic environments but instead tends to adsorb onto organic particles and to bioconcentrate in organisms. As is typical with other lipophilic environmental toxicants, highest concentrations of DDT are observed in organisms at the top of the food web. In some studies, levels as high as 10 to 20 ppm were measured in some seabirds, and high levels have also been found in larger fish and marine mammals. While DDT is no longer used in the U.S., its use continues in other parts of the world, and residues have been found even in Antarctic birds.

DDT
see also:
Organochlorines   *Appendix, p. 241*

Although mammalian toxicity is relatively low (oral LD_{50} of around 200 mg/kg) DDT is, of course, toxic to many insect species including flies, beetles, and mosquitoes (the vector for the malaria-causing organism *Plasmodium*). For insects, though, pesticides are just another selection pressure. Because insects are rapidly reproducing r strategists, insect populations can adapt very quickly to the presence of pesticides through the evolution of resistant populations. Fish, also,

TABLE 1   Organochlorine Insecticides

Dichlorodiphenylethanes

DDT
Methoxychlor

Cyclodienes

Chlordane
Heptachlor
Aldrin
Dieldrin

Hexachlorocyclohexanes

Lindane

are affected, with the young of many species (such as salmon, for example) being particularly sensitive. While there is evidence that fish may suffer from behavioral and reproductive changes following exposure to DDT, the effects of DDT on fish populations do seem to be reversible, however. DDT is also toxic to several species of algae.

The most significant effects of DDT on wildlife are on birds of prey, especially those species which prey on fish. As K strategists, large birds are slower to reproduce and thus slower to develop adaptive mutations. The combination of these slow reproductive rates with the tendency of DDT to bioaccumulate have led to severe impacts on bird populations. Populations of grebes, bald eagles, peregrine falcons, and osprey have all reportedly been affected by DDT. DDT causes changes in reproduction characterized by alterations in mating and parental behavior, decreases in number of eggs laid, decreases in number of eggs successfully hatched (due at least in part to decreased eggshell thickness), and increased mortality rates among chicks. Although the survival of many populations in the U.S. was threatened, some are now recovering following the ban on DDT use here first by Wisconsin and Michigan and then by the EPA.

Two other major classes of insecticides (which share a basic mechanism of action) are the *organophosphates* and *carbamates* (Table 2). These are the current insecticides of choice for many uses, because they are relatively nonpersistent (with half lives measured in weeks rather than years) and are considerably more water soluble than the organochlorines. Organophosphates tend to be more toxic to invertebrates than

ORGANOPHOSPHATES
see also:
Biotransformation ***Ch. 2 p. 24***
Cellular sites of action ***Ch. 4, p. 40***
Neurotoxicology ***Ch. 9, pp. 130, 137***
Water pollution ***Ch. 15, p. 217***
Organophosphates ***Appendix, p. 242***

CARBAMATES
see also:
Carbamates ***Appendix, p. 235***

TABLE 2 Other Insecticides

Organophosphates
Parathion
Fenitrothion
Malathion
Carbamates
Carbaryl
Aminocarb
Carbofuran
Pyrethroids
Allethrin

to fish. For example, the 96 hour LC_{50} for methyl parathion ranges around 10 $\mu g/l$ for invertebrates as compared to over 5000 $\mu g/l$ for fish.

The *pyrethroids* are another class of insecticides (Table 2). These compounds have low persistence, partially due to rapid metabolism and detoxification by cytochrome P450 systems, and bind so strongly to soil particles that availability to nontarget organisms is relatively low, although they are toxic to fish in the low parts per billion range.

Herbicides are often used to control aquatic plants and algal growth. Some common herbicides which are potential pollutants are listed in Table 3. Among the most widely used herbicides are the chlorphenoxy acids *2,4-dichlorophe-noxyacetic acid (2,4-D)* and *2,4,5-trichlorophenoxyacetic acid (2,4,5-T)*.

These compounds typically provide fewer water pollution problems than DDT for several reasons: (1) their much higher water solubility encourages dilution rather than bioconcentration; and (2) their residence times in the environment are much shorter, on the order of

---

2,4-D, 2,4,5-T
see also:
   Renal toxicicology   *Ch. 11, p. 116*
   2,4-D, 2,4,5-T   *Appendix, p. 237*

---

weeks rather than years. Also, LD_{50}s for most species are high (on the order of several hundred mg/kg). Many of the reported adverse effects (such as reproductive and teratogenic effects and immunosuppression) related to exposure to these compounds may instead be due to a contami-nant, *2,3,7,8-tetra-chlorodibenzo-p-dioxin (TCDD)*. The range of LD_{50}s for TCDD is much, much lower, with values for some species of less than one microgram/kilogram. Because of its low solubility, and its tendency to bind tightly to soils, TCDD is, however, rarely detected in water.

2,3,7,8-TCDD
see also:
   Biotransformation   *Ch. 3, p. 28*
   Carcinogenesis   *Ch. 5, p. 59*
   Immunotoxicology   *Ch. 12, p. 179*
   TCDD   *Appendix, p. 245*

PARAQUAT
see also:
   Respiratory
      toxicology   *Ch. 7, p. 97*
   Paraquat   *Appendix, p. 243*

A different class of herbicide includes the bipyridyl herbicides, *paraquat* and *diquat*. Diquat is commonly applied to aquatic environments, and has an LD_{50} of around 100 to 200 mg/kg in mammalian species, and causes free-radical induced damage to liver and kidney (in contrast to paraquat, which accumulates in and preferen-

TABLE 3   Herbicides

Chlorphenoxy Acids

2,4-D
2,4,5-T

Bipyridals

Paraquat
Diquat

tially affects the lung). Both these compounds bind tightly to soils and have very long half lives (more than 5 years).

Finally, two organometallic compounds are frequently used for pest control in aquatic environments: (1) copper sulfate—a commonly used algicide; and (2) tributyltin—a antifoulant commonly used to control growth of barnacles and other organisms on the hulls of ships. The toxicity of these compounds will be discussed under the section on metals.

Other Organic Compounds

Pollution by *plastics* has become a significant problem, primarily because of the chemical stability of most plastics. Every year tons of plastic trash are dumped into bodies of water where it floats free or washes up onto beaches and shores. Problems arise particularly in the ocean, where buoyant plastic trash such as plastic netting, fishing line, and six-pack rings entangle marine birds, reptiles, fish, and mammals. Some studies estimate, for example, that tens of thousands of seals are killed each year by plastic debris, and even whales may be fatally tied up in discarded netting. Plastic may also be mistaken for food and consumed by these animals, blocking and causing irritation of the gastrointestinal tract.

Another group of organic compounds of particular concern are the *trihalomethanes* (chloroform, bromodichloromethane, and dibromochloromethane). Some of these compounds appear naturally in water, while others are thought to be produced by reaction of chlorine (added as a disinfectant) with organic matter in the water. Formation of trihalomethanes is limited if chlorine is added as the final step in water treatment (after most organic compounds have already been removed). The presence of these compounds in drinking water has been associated with an increased risk of several types of cancer.

A group of synthetic organic chemicals, the *polychlorinated biphenyls* (*PCBs*) have been linked to several ecological and health-related effects. These highly lipophilic, persistent compounds are primarily used as insulating material in electrical components, and enter the water supply through discharge of industrial effluents and leaching from landfills and hazardous

PCBS

see also:

Immunotoxicology   *Ch. 12, p. 179*
PCBs   *Appendix, p. 243*

waste dumps. Also, because very high temperatures are required to destroy these compounds, incomplete incineration may also lead to their release. One of many areas which has been polluted with PCBs is the upper Hudson River in NY, where two factories which manufactured capacitors dumped PCBs into the river for more than 30 years.

Due to their lipophilicity and persistence, PCBs bioaccumulate, and can be found in aquatic organisms in virtually all parts of the world. Levels of PCBs in some species of fish collected from the upper Hudson in 1977 averaged as high as 6000 μg/g. The levels of PCBs in this ecosystem are now declining (slowly) due to slowing of rate of discharge, dredging and removal of some contaminated sediments, and the gradual degradation of the compounds.

PCBs are more toxic to fish than to birds or mammals, and have been found to interfere with reproductive function in a number of different species. PCBs lead to induction of cytochrome P450 in mammals, and have been reported to cause liver cancer in rats. In addition, they are immunosuppressants.

INORGANIC POLLUTANTS

Phosphorus and Nitrogen

Phosphorus and sometimes *nitrogen* are what is known as *limiting nutrients*, meaning that they are among the first necessary nutrients to become depleted and thus to limit the rate of growth of a plant population. These two essential nutrients occur in many chemical forms. Most of the available phosphorus in aquatic environments is in the form of *phosphate* (PO_4^{3-}). Primary forms of nitrogen include *nitrate* (NO_3) or *ammonium ion* (NH_4^+). When human activities around a body of water result in the addition of phosphorus and nitrogen, rapid bursts of algal and plant growth (sometimes called blooms) can occur. Lakes are particularly susceptible. Algae levels increase, activity of decomposers must increase (to breakdown dead algae), and as a result oxygen levels become depleted (affecting many species of fish). This input of additional nutrients and the resulting ecological changes is called *cultural eutrophication*.

CULTURAL EUTROPHICATION
see also:
Ecological toxicology   Ch. 13, p. 195

There are many activities which can contribute to cultural eutrophication. Municipal waste waters account for most of the input, carrying nitrogen and phosphorus-rich sewage as well as phosphates from detergents (phosphates are used in detergents to bind ions which may interfere in the cleaning process). Agricultural runoff may also contain phosphates and nitrates leached from the soil following fertilizer application.

One of the areas in the U.S. which has suffered from eutrophication is the Great Lakes. Lake Erie, in particular, has been affected as a result of the many urban and agricultural activities on its shores. At one point, one region of Lake Erie had phosphorus concentrations that were eight times that of the much less affected Lake Superior. Algae levels increased, mayfly larvae and other benthic insects disappeared, and populations of trout and whitefish declined.

Cultural eutrophication is fortunately reversible with time. Reduction of phosphate and nitrate input will eventually restore lakes to their original, more oligotrophic condition. Recently, due to the Great Lakes Water Quality Agreement signed by the U.S. and Canada, phosphorus input into Lake Erie has decreased, and algal growth has dramatically declined. Oxygen levels near the bottom of the lake also appear to have improved.

The presence of nitrates in drinking water has also been associated with a human health problem called *methemoglobinemia*. In this condition, nitrates are converted in the body to nitrites, which oxidize hemoglobin and prevent the molecule from carrying oxygen. Infants are particularly susceptible.

NITRATES
see also:
Cellular sites	*Ch. 4, p. 54*
Cardiovascular	
toxicology	*Ch. 8, pp. 111, 115*
Nitrates	*Appendix, p. 240*

Metals

Although *metals* are normally present in the environment, human activities may increase metal concentrations in aquatic environments to levels which may be hazardous to ecological systems or human health. Metals interact with water and other compounds in a complicated manner, with each metal forming many different *species*, or chemical forms, depending on conditions. Metals can be found in water as the *free metal ion*, or combined with chloride or a variety of other anions to form an *ion pair*. Metals also bind to both small and large organic molecules. Small organometallic molecules are frequently soluble in water, while the larger complexes formed by association of metals with large organic components of soils and sediments are usually not. Factors such as pH and *hardness* (the concentration of calcium, magnesium, and other cations in the solution) can affect the relative concentrations of different species of a metal.

Speciation of metals is often key in determining effects of metals in an aquatic environment, as different species of the same metal may vary widely in toxicity. For example, some studies have found that copper carbonate ($CuCO_3$) is much less toxic to trout than copper hydroxide ($Cu(OH)_2$) or copper ion (Cu^{2+}). Also, complexation with organic matter generally lowers toxicity by making the metal less available for absorption by organisms. Bioaccumulation of metals does occur, particularly in plants. Organisms do have the potential to metabolize some metals, thus altering their chemical species and genes for copper resistance have evolved in plant pathogenic bacteria selected by agricultural use of copper bactericides, suggesting novel means of bioremediation.

LEAD
see also:
Reproductive toxicology	***Ch. 6, p. 75***
Cardiovascular toxicology	***Ch. 8, p. 114***
Immunotoxicology	***Ch. 12, p. 180***
Neurotoxicology	***Ch. 9, p. 140, 143***
Lead	***Appendix, p. 239***

One metal with toxic potential is *lead*. Lead enters lakes and streams when it leaches from soils as a component of runoff. It then tends to accumulate in sediments, with freshwater levels generally only reaching a few micrograms per liter. Lead is a much more significant problem in drinking water, where it may leach from lead pipes or solder and reach concentrations of 50 μg/l or higher. Lead produces neurological and hematological effects.

CADMIUM
see also:
Reproductive toxicology	***Ch. 6, p. 75***
Cardiovascular toxicology	***Ch. 8, p. 111***
Renal toxicology	***Ch. 11, p. 165***
Cadmium	***Appendix, p. 235***

Many of the various species of *cadmium* are quite soluble in water, and also tend to bioaccumulate (particularly in shellfish, but also in fish and plants). Cadmium's potential as a toxic water pollutant was demonstrated in Japan, in areas where water from the Jinzu River in Toyama Prefecture, Honshu was used to irrigate rice fields. Many people in this area, particularly older women, suffered from a disease they called "itai-itai" or "ouch ouch" because of the severe bone pain that accompanied it. Itai-itai was characterized by severe osteoporosis and kidney dysfunction. The river in the affected area was highly polluted by a mining operation upstream which was discharging tailings that were contaminated with cadmium (among other metals). Cadmium bioaccumulated to high levels in rice from the irrigated fields, and consequently in the people who consumed the rice. Levels of cadmium and other metals in the tissues of afflicted persons were found to be as high as several parts per thousand, confirming metal pollution as the cause.

MERCURY
see also:
Reproductive toxicology	***Ch. 6, p. 75***
Neurotoxicology	***Ch. 9, p. 142***
Renal toxicology	***Ch. 11, p. 162***
Mercury	***Appendix, p. 239***

A second incident in Japan involved pollution by another heavy metal, *mercury*. Mercury which was released into Minamata Bay in Kumamoto Prefecture, Kyushu by a plastics manufacturer was methylated by microorganisms in the bay to form *methylmercury*, a neurotoxicant. Bioconcentration occurred, and effects were seen in organisms near the top of the food chain. Large fish were found dead in the bay, seabirds fell into the water, and the cats living in villages around the bay began to stagger around (this lead to the nickname of "dancing cat disease" for the condition). And, because the inhabitants of bayside villages derived most of their food from the bay, they too were affected.

Another organometal which is a water pollutant is the compound *tributyltin* (*TBT*). This compound is used to kill barnacles, mussels, and other organisms which attach themselves to the hulls of ships. Usually, TBT is incorporated into paint, which releases the chemical gradually. Unfortunately, many marine species such as oysters are extremely sensitive to TBT, with some species showing effects (shell malformations, reproductive effects) at levels as low as a few parts per billion. This has led to more stringent regulation, and in some cases banning of TBT use.

Zinc, although an essential trace element, can produce toxicity through interference with absorption of copper and iron, leading to anemia. Zinc can also cause necrosis of gill tissues. Increased levels of zinc may,

---

METALLOTHIONEIN
see also:
   Toxicokinetics   *Ch. 2, p. 15*

---

however, protect against cadmium poisoning, perhaps through induction of the cadmium and zinc binding enzyme metallothionein. High concentrations of *copper* (which is often used as an algicide) can lead to accumulation of the metal in the liver (an effect seen in both mammals and fish).

OTHER POLLUTANTS

Biological agents frequently enter water systems when sewage is inadequately treated. This is particularly a problem in less developed countries where water treatment systems are rarely adequate. Contact with the contaminated water through swimming, drinking, or eating contaminated fish or shellfish can then lead to infection. Diseases which can spread in this manner include bacterial infections such as *cholera* and *typhoid*, as well as diseases caused by protozoans such as *amoebic dysentery*.

When sediment is carried off from land into water, it becomes *suspended matter*. Suspended matter can block sunlight, and thus prevent photosynthesis. And, because many sediment particles contain organic matter, suspended matter can contribute to the problem of eutrophication.

Thermal pollution is a problem associated most frequently with power plants. These plants bring in cool water from a nearby ocean, lake, or stream, and then discharge it at a higher temperature. The higher the temperature and the greater the volume of the discharged water, the more significant the problem is likely to be. Warm water holds less dissolved oxygen than cooler water, and at the same time the increased temperature causes an increase in body temperature and thus rates of cellular respiration for many aquatic organisms. The increased oxygen requirements associated with the changes in respiration combine with the lower availability of oxygen to produce oxygen deprivation.

REGULATION AND CONTROL OF WATER POLLUTION

Water pollution in the U.S. is regulated by two major laws: the Clean Water Act (originally written in 1972 and most recently reauthorized as the Water Quality Act of 1987) and the Safe Drinking Water Act written in 1974. The Clean Water Act and its reauthorizations require industries to pretreat wastes before discharge into municipal water systems, and require permits for discharges into navigable waters. In addition, federal financial support is provided for construction of better water treatment facilities. The Safe Drinking Water Act requires the establishment of maximum acceptable levels for pollutants (maximum contaminant levels or MCLs) in drinking water. The process, however, is slow, and standards have not been set for all chemicals known or suspected to be a problem. A general wastewater treatment scheme is shown in Figure 1.

WASTE WATER TREATMENT

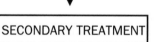

PRIMARY TREATMENT

screens and filters remove solid materials
(which are then sent to sanitary landfill)

↓

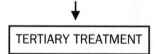

SECONDARY TREATMENT

small particles settle out in settling tanks
(the sludge which results from this
step must then be disposed of by
incineration, digestion, or burial)
in an aeration tank, aserobic bacteria are then
allowed to digest the remaining organic materials
(the bacteria are then allowed to settle
out and are added to the sludge)

↓

TERTIARY TREATMENT

the removal of phosphorus, nitrogen, metals, and
other pollutants requires additional special treatments

Figure 1   Wastewater treatment.

REFERENCES

Borgmann, U., Metal speciation and toxicity of free metal ions to aquatic biota, in *Aquatic Toxicology*, Nriagu, J. O., Ed., John Wiley & Sons, New York, 1983, chap. 2.

Brown, M. P., Werner, M. B., Sloan, R. J., and Simpson, K. W., Polychlorinated biphenyls in the Hudson River, *Environ. Sci. Technol.*, 19, 1985.

Cherfas, J., The fringe of the ocean—under siege from land, *Science*, 248, 163, 1990.

Connell, D. W. and Miller, G. J., *Chemistry and Ecotoxicology of Pollution*, John Wiley & Sons, New York, 1984, chaps. 5, 6, 12.

DePinto, J. V., Young, T. C., and McIlroy, L. M., Great Lakes water quality improvement, *Environ. Sci. Technol.*, 20, 752, 1986.

Ecobichon, D. J., Toxic effects of pesticides, in *Casarett and Doull's Toxicology*, Amdur, M. O., Doull, J., and Klaassen, C. D., Eds., Pergamon Press, New York, 1991, chap. 18.

Freedman, B., *Environmental Ecology*, Academic Press, San Diego, CA, 1989, chap. 6.

Heckman, C. W., Reactions of aquatic ecosystems to pesticides, in *Aquatic Toxicology*, Nriagu, J. O., Ed., John Wiley & Sons, New York, 1983, chap. 12.

Holloway, M., Soiled shores, *Sci. Am.*, Oct. 1991, 102.

Huggett, R. J., Unger, M. A., Seligman, P. F., and Valkirs, A. O., The marine biocide tributyltin, *Environ. Sci. Technol.* 26, 232, 1992.

Laxen, D. P. H., The chemistry of metal pollutants in water, in *Pollution: Causes, Effects, and Control*, Hasrrison, R. M., Ed., Royal Society of Chemistry, London, 1982, chap. 6.

Leland, H. V. and Kuwabara, J. S., Trace metals, in *Fundamentals of Aquatic Toxicology*, Rand, G. M. and Petrocelli, S. R., Eds., Hemisphere, Washington, DC, 1985, chap. 13.

Levy, E. M., Oil pollution in the world's oceans, *Ambio*, 13, 226, 1984.

Makarewicz, J. C. and Bertram, P., Evidence for the restoration of the Lake Erie ecosystem, *Bioscience*, 41, 216, 1991.

Maurits la Riviere, J. W., Threats to the world's water, *Sci. Am.*, Sept., 1989, 80.

Menzer, R. E., Water and soil pollutants, in *Casarett and Doull's Toxicology*, Amdur, M. O., Doull, J., and Klaassen, C. D., Eds., Pergamon Press, New York, 1991, chap. 26.

Nimmo, D. R., Pesticides, in *Fundamentals of Aquatic Toxicology*, Rand, G. M. and Petrocelli, S. R., Eds., Hemisphere, Washington, DC, 1985, chap. 12.

Stumm, W., Water, an endangered ecosystem, *Ambio*, 15, 201, 1986.

Weisskopf, M., Plastic reaps a grim harvest in the oceans of the world, *Smithsonian*, 18, 59, 1988.

16 TOXIC WASTES

SOURCES OF WASTES

One serious consequence of the industrial revolution and modern development has been the generation of toxic waste materials. Toxic wastes are generated by many activities in the modern society, including manufacturing and other industrial processes, and also in the consumption or utilization of manufactured goods. While *toxicity* of waste substances can be estimated by a median lethal dose study or similar experiment, estimating the actual *hazard* posed by a waste involves estimating not only intrinsic toxicity of the substance, but also factors such as the likelihood that exposure to the substance will occur. *Toxic waste*, when handled or disposed in such a way as to threaten public health or the environment, can be considered *hazardous waste*.

Generators of hazardous waste can be found in every segment of society. Activities which generate hazardous wastes include: manufacturing, mining, defense (weapons manufacture), agriculture, utility company operations (power plants), small business operations (dry cleaners, paint shops, automobile service, etc.), hospital operations, laboratory research, and even household and municipal activities.

CATEGORIES OF WASTE

The great majority of hazardous waste is produced by large generators in manufacturing, mining, and the military. These sources discard wastes containing toxicants such as *organic solvents*, *polycyclic aromatic hydrocarbons*, *pesticides*, and *heavy metals*. In a survey of 1189 sites the most commonly found solvents included 1,1,2-trichloroethylene (found in 401 sites), toluene (found in 281 sites), and benzene (found in 249 sites). Polycyclic aromatic hydrocarbons found included naphthalene (60 sites), phenanthrene (41 sites), and benzo[a]pyrene (37 sites). Among the many toxic metals founds were lead (395 sites), chromium (395 sites), and arsenic (187 sites). Polychlorinated biphenyls were found in 185 sites and the chlorinated organic insecticides DDT and chlordane were found in 50 and 33 sites, respectively. Some Department of Energy sites hold radioactive plutonium, cesium, and uranium in an extremely toxic sludge with no known means of remediation.

Household hazardous waste disposal is also a growing problem. Organic solvents are used in every household; there is methanol or phenol in many bathroom cleaning agents, chloroform in some toothpastes, and ethyl acetate in fingernail polish. Inorganic cleaning agents include sodium hypochlorite in bleach and ammonium hydroxide in household ammonia. An increasing number of household and personal appliances are powered by small alkaline nickel and cadmium batteries which are often disposed with garbage. Household paints and home and garden pesticides are used in large volumes and unused portions often accumulate until they become outdated and thus considered waste. Considered cumulatively, a community of many consuming households may generate a considerable volume of toxic waste and should attempt to manage that waste just as a manufacturing plant must, by law, manage its hazardous waste.

LEGISLATION CONCERNING HAZARDOUS WASTE

The first-generation solution to industrial and municipal waste was to bury it underground or at sea. Such dumping has resulted in landfills which are now slowly leaking undefined mixtures into groundwater and a buildup of waste materials contaminating the oceans, and in some cases, washing back onshore. Public awareness of hazardous waste was heightened by several epidemiological studies indicating increased risks of disease in persons residing near large, industrial hazardous waste dumping sites. It became clear that, from an environmental perspective, disposal is only temporary because, in many situations, the air, surface water, or groundwater can easily become contaminated from the disposed hazardous waste in the future. As a result of these concerns, legislation has been passed which defines hazardous waste and requires the use of approved disposal methods.

In the U.S., legislation has addressed hazardous waste so that it is regulated by the Environmental Protection Agency. The *Resource Conservation and Recovery Act of 1976* (*RCRA*) with its *Hazardous and Solid Waste Amendments of 1984* established requirement for management of hazardous waste generated through many activities (although some sources were exempted).

One major contribution of RCRA was the definition of *hazardous waste* as ignitable, corrosive, reactive, or toxic substances. All "solid" (defined in the act as solid, liquid, semisolid, or gas in a container) hazardous waste was to be treated prior to being placed in specially constructed, secure landfills. The act exempted industrial effluent and irrigation return flows (which are regulated under the *Clean Water Act*), nuclear waste (regulated under the *Atomic Energy Act*), household waste, coal combustion waste, agricultural fertilizers, petrochemical drilling muds, some mining wastes, and cement kiln dust. However, these categories may be added by future amendments.

Remedial action to prevent environmental damage from existing hazardous waste dump sites was directed under the *Comprehensive Environmental Response and Recovery Act of 1980 (CERCLA)*, also known as "*Superfund.*" Under the *Superfund Amendments and Reauthorization Act of 1986*, the most threatening dump sites were identified and ranked in priority for remediation. In 1991, the *National Priorities List* included 1189 uncontrolled hazardous waste sites eligible for remedial action by the federal government. These included 116 federal sites, mostly nuclear (Department of Energy) or defense facilities, and 231 municipal landfill sites. These sites also included commercial or industrial landfills and surface impoundments (evaporation ponds), and chemical manufacturing or processing areas filled with containers or drums. Many sites were associated with electroplating (chromium, copper, mercury), military testing and ordnance (chemical warfare agents, explosives), wood preserving (pentachlorophenol), waste oil processing (lead, benzene, etc.), ore processing (fluoride, arsenic, etc.), battery recycling (lead, cadmium), and incineration (metals, PAHs, PCBs). The site encompassing the largest surface area was the Anaconda, MI, smetter, which generated airborne particles of arsenicals during several decades of silver, copper, and manganese ore processing.

Sites on the National Priorities List were found throughout the U.S., but tended to cluster around major cities. There were 204 sites in New York and New Jersey (EPA Region 2), and 37% of the sites were in the combined EPA regions 1, 2, and 3, which encompass the 13 northeastern states from Maine to Virginia. There were also 260 sites listed in the 6 states of EPA region 5, which border the Great Lakes. Therefore 57.7% of the total sites were in 19 states of the northeast and upper Midwest.

Candidate sites for the National Priorities List of 1991 were rated by a Hazard Ranking System for the relative threat to human health or the environment; and the 1189 considered most hazardous were listed. The most threatening nonfederal sites were Lipari Landfill, Pitman, NJ; Tybouts Corner Landfill, New Castle County, DE; Bruin Lagoon, Bruin Borough, PA, Helen Kramer Landfill, Mantua Township, NJ; and Industri-Plex, Woburn, MA. The highest ranking federal sites were two areas of the Hanford Nuclear Reservation, WA; Rocky Flats Plant, Golden, CO; Riverbank Army Ammunition Plant, CA; Cal West Metals, Lemitar, NM; and Weldon Spring Quarry, St. Charles County, MO.

Following development of the National Priorities List, the next step was to begin to take action for remediation of those sites. Funding for contracted remediatory projects is provided by a trust fund which is administered by the EPA. The trust fund is generated by a tax on manufacturers, cost recovery through litigation, federal appropriation, and interest.

Many problems have complicated the cleanup task, such as the fact that leaking containers at hundreds of sites have deteriorated so badly that it has become difficult to stabilize the site without causing more leakage. Also, these conditions tend to produce mixtures of diverse organic and inorganic toxic compounds which present complex technical difficulties in designing detoxication strategies. Political pressures and diversity of opinion over treatment strategies have also led to delays.

Because of the need for many preliminary investigations and plans to be made for each site in order to deal with these factors, the cleanup rates have been very slow. Also, the most hazardous (and therefore the most complex) sites have required the most planning, and thus have not necessarily been the first to be cleaned. This slowness of action has generated a great deal of criticism for the EPA and the program as a whole.

A new, more detailed Hazard Ranking System has been developed and the National Priorities List is updated annually. As of 1994, there are 1286 sites on the National Priorities List. Remediation has been completed to the point of formal deletion of approximately 57 sites from the original list. Another 235 sites are in the construction/completion stage meaning that they are in active remediation, while most of the remaining sites are in some phase of investigation, construction, or remediation.

MANAGEMENT OF WASTE

A plan for the management of hazardous waste may employ various techniques which may be classified into the following categories: *reducing the volume generated*, *recycling*, *treatment*, and *storage*. Storage of an accumulating volume of hazardous waste, however, must be viewed as the least desirable way to manage the problem, and should be considered as a temporary approach while other ways are found to eliminate the hazardous waste.

Reducing the Volume Generated

Industry in the U.S. generates about 10 billion tons of industrial wastes annually. Out of this amount, about 275 million tons are hazardous wastes. Manufacturing of paints, dyes, polymers, plastics, and high technology items, such as computer circuit boards and semiconductors, generate toxic wastes from the reactants in their synthesis and the solvents used in their manufacture.

Reducing the volume of hazardous waste is becoming a major emphasis in industry as a result of increasing treatment and disposal costs. Waste minimization programs involve quantification of the waste produced, identification of the source of waste in the process, and engineering to improve the efficiency of the manufacturing process, or to substitute less toxic compounds for the endproduct and for the intermediates in the process stream. Finding alternatives to those products generating toxic waste is the ounce of prevention which, in this case, is worth much more than a pound of cure. Alternatives have been found for PCBs, DDT, ozone-depleting chlorofluorocarbons, and other environmental pollutants.

Recycling

A large industry has developed for the recycling of waste, including toxic substances. For example, industrial process and cleaning solvents are now routinely recycled so that approximately two thirds of solvent used is recovered. Solvent recycling is accomplished by sequential settling, filtering, and distillation—so it is a relatively simple process. Rather than disposal of the contaminated solvent, contaminants collected as filter cake and still bottoms are treated for detoxication or decomposed, and recycled solvent is obtained at high yield.

Treatment

Detoxication is the reduction of toxicity of waste through physical, chemical, or biological treatment. Ultraviolet irradiation in methanol is used to detoxify TCDD and pesticides by dechlorination. In an aqueous stream containing hazardous waste, chemical oxidation, reduction, or hydrolysis may be used to detoxify the waste. In some cases separation of the hazardous waste from the liquid process or waste stream may be accomplished by precipitation, centrifugation, or filtration. This results in a concentrated cake or solid which can be collected for detoxication. Separation depends on the chemical characteristic of the waste constituents. Useful filtration matrices include silica for organic solvent streams, ion exchange resins, and activated carbon.

Biodegradation has the advantage of being inexpensive because microorganisms are used to degrade the waste. Enzymes within or secreted from the microorganism catalyze detoxication reactions such as hydrolysis, oxidation, or reduction. Recent advances in biotechnology have succeeded in engineering microorganisms for more efficient waste degradation. The treatment of existing toxic waste sites by this technique is known as *bioremediation*.

Incineration is the burning of waste composed of organic compounds in the presence of oxygen at temperatures of up to about 1500°C. High temperature combustion will detoxify many toxic, organic compounds by oxidation to carbon dioxide and water. As the waste burns, the heat evolved may be used for the manufacturing process or for some other purpose. Incineration does not produce detoxication of all types of hazardous wastes, and may even produce added toxic oxides as the waste is oxidized. Also, incineration at reduced temperature may simply volatilize the waste. For these reasons, incineration smoke may be toxic and, if so, must be scrubbed before entering the atmosphere. In addition, the

Supreme Court has recently ruled that ash from municipal incinerators must be regulated as potentially hazardous waste.

Pyrolysis is a more universally detoxicative process which employs extremely high heat, like in an iron smelter, to decompose organic and inorganic toxic compounds to elemental form. This process is expensive, energy consuming, and not commonly available; however, new companies specializing in this process are likely to grow rapidly, thus lowering the costs somewhat. This process is most elegant because it is the simplification of toxic wastes to the elements from which they originated.

Monitored Storage

Storage of hazardous waste in secure landfills is considered by EPA as a temporary approach while other ways are found to eliminate the hazardous waste. Under the Resource Conservation and Recovery Act, secure landfills must meet construction standards and disposal must be preceded by characterization and treatment of the waste.

EPA regulations include Land Disposal Restrictions which state that all hazardous waste must be treated to meet Best Demonstrated Achievable Technology prior to land disposal. These regulations require measuring the concentrations of waste constituents by approved test methods before or after a Toxicity Characteristic Leaching Procedure which simulates leaching of the constituents from the solid matrix.

Secure landfills must be constructed with liners to prevent leaching down to the groundwater. They must also have a drainage system above the liner to collect leaking waste into a holding system. Secure landfills must also have adjacent monitoring wells to test for contamination of the surrounding area.

REFERENCES

Cashman, J. R., *Management of Hazardous Waste*, Technomic Pub. Co., Inc., Lancaster, PA, 1986.

Englande, A. J. J. & Eckenfelder, W. W. J., Toxic waste management in the chemical and petrochemical industries, in *IAWPRC 2nd Intern'l Conf. Waste Manag. Chem. Petrochem. Indust., Water Sci. Technol.*, 25, 286, 1991.

Environmental Protection Agency, National priorities list for uncontrolled hazardous waste sites. *Fed. Reg.*, 59, 27989, 1994.

Environmental Protection Agency, National priorities list under the original hazard ranking system 1981–1991 (*Fact Book No. 9320.7-08, EPA 540-R-93-079*), EPA Office of Solid Waste and Emergency Response, 1993.

Epstein, S. S., Brown, L. O., and Pope, C., *Hazardous Waste in America*, San Francisco, Sierra Club Books, CA, 1982, 593.

Turner, S. M., Hazardous waste management, *Information Pamphlet*, American Chemical Society, 1992.

APPENDIX / List of Selected Toxicants

NAME: **Acetaminophen**
CHEMICAL FORMULA: p-hydroxyacetanilide $C_8H_9NO_2$
PHYSICAL PROPERTIES: crystals
SOURCES AND USES: Synthetic compound used to treat headache, inflammation, fever
TOXICITY: LD_{50} (mice, oral) 338 mg/kg
SEE ALSO: Hepatotoxicity Ch. 10, p. 154

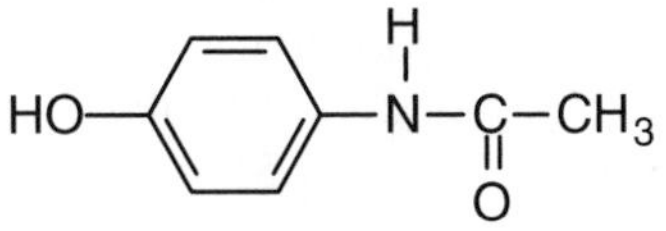

acetaminophen

NAME: **Aflatoxins**
CHEMICAL FORMULA: Aflatoxin B_1 (2,3,6aα, 9aα-Tetrahydro-4-methoxy-cyclopenta [c]furo[3′,2′:4,5]furo[2,3-h][1]benzopyran-1,11-dione) $C_{17}H_{12}O_6$
PHYSICAL PROPERTIES: crystals
SOURCES AND USES: Produced by *Aspergillus sp.* (fungi), can contaminate food products under proper conditions
TOXICITY: Hepatotoxicants, carcinogens. LD_{50} (mouse, ip) 9.5 mg/kg
SEE ALSO: Hepatotoxicity Ch. 10, p. 156

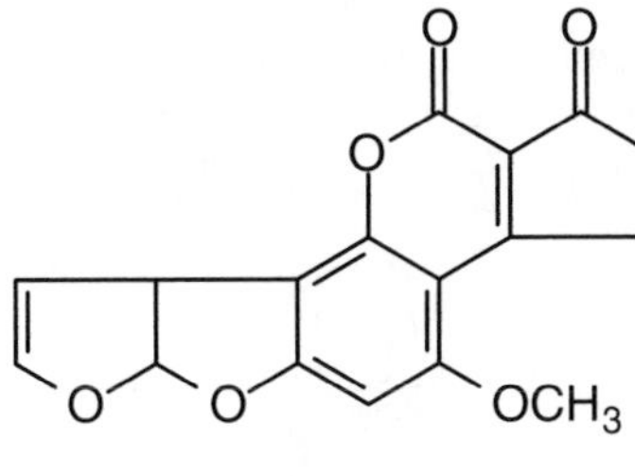

aflatoxin B_1

NAME: **Arsenic**
CHEMICAL FORMULA: As
PHYSICAL PROPERTIES: gray-black, metallic crystal. Many different species, most toxic
SOURCES AND USES: Naturally occurring element, used in manufacture of glass, metal working; contaminant of precious metal ore.
TOXICITY: Gastrointestinal irritant, nephrotoxicant, hepatotoxicant. LD_{50} arsenic trioxide, (mouse, oral) 39.4 mg/kg
SEE ALSO: Toxic waste   Ch. 16. p. 228

$$As_2O_3$$

arsenic trioxide (arsenous acid)

NAME: **Asbestos**
CHEMICAL FORMULA: chrysotile (the most common form of asbestos) $Mg_6(Si_4O_{10})(OH)_8$
PHYSICAL PROPERTIES: Fibrous silicate
SOURCE AND USES: Naturally occurring, used as a heat and fire-resistant material.
TOXICITY: Respiratory toxicant, carcinogen
SEE ALSO: Respiratory toxicology   Ch. 7, p. 99

$$[Mg_6(Si_4O_{10})(OH)_8]$$

asbestos (chrysotile)

NAME: **Benzene**
CHEMICAL FORMULA: C_6H_6
PHYSICAL PROPERTIES: Clear, colorless, flammable liquid
SOURCE AND USES: Can be purified from coal, or synthesized. Used in manufacture of many compounds.
TOXICITY: Acute exposures lead to nervous system depression, with an LD_{50} (rat, oral) of 3.8 ml/kg. Chronic exposure has been associated with bone marrow depression and leukemia.
SEE ALSO: Cardiovascular toxicology   Ch. 8, p. 113
                   Immunotoxicology   Ch. 12, p. 170

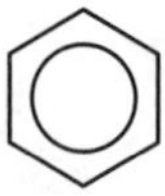

benzene

NAME: **Cadmium**
CHEMICAL FORMULA: Cd
PHYSICAL PROPERTIES: Heavy metal
SOURCE AND USES: Naturally occurring, used in making of metal alloys, batteries, and other products.
TOXICITY: Reproductive toxicant, cardiovascular toxicant, renal toxicant
SEE ALSO: Reproductive toxicology Ch. 6, p. 75
Cardiovascular toxicology Ch. 8, p. 111
Renal toxicology Ch. 11, p. 165
Water pollution Ch. 15, p. 232

Cd

cadmium

NAME: **Carbamate pesticides**
CHEMICAL FORMULA: Carbaryl (1-Naphthalenol methylcarbamate) $C_{12}H_{11}NO_2$ Aldicarb (2-Methyl-2(methylthio)propanal O- [(methylamino)carbonyl]oxime) $C_7H_{14}N_2O_2S$
PHYSICAL PROPERTIES: Crystals
SOURCES AND USES: Synthetic pesticides; insecticides
TOXICITY: Neurotoxicity. LD_{50} carbaryl (rat, oral) 250 mg/kg; aldicarb (rat, oral) 1 mg/kg
SEE ALSO: Water pollution Ch. 15, p. 217

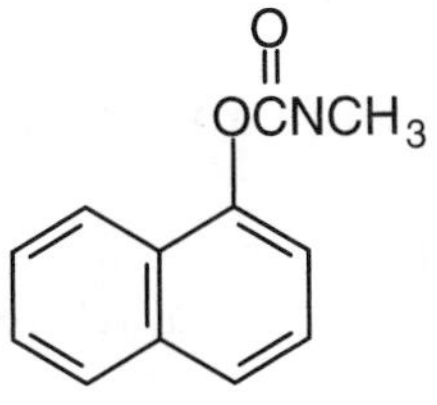

carbaryl
(Sevin®)

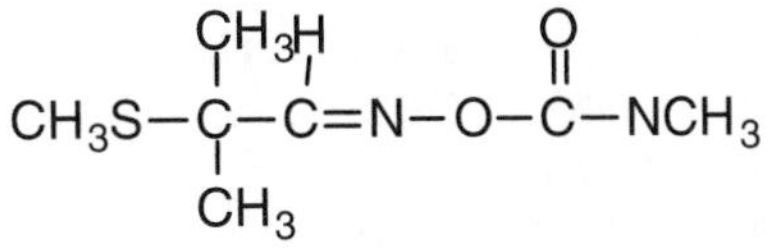

aldicarb

NAME: **Carbon disulfide**
CHEMICAL FORMULA: CS_2
PHYSICAL PROPERTIES: Flammable liquid
SOURCE AND USES: Synthesized. Used in manufacture of rayon, and as cleaning solvent.

TOXICITY: Cardiovascular toxicant, neurotoxicant
SEE ALSO: Cardiovascular toxicology   Ch. 8, p. 110
             Neurotoxicology   Ch. 9, p. 138

$$CS_2$$

carbon disulfide

NAME: **Carbon monoxide**
CHEMICAL FORMULA: CO
PHYSICAL PROPERTIES: colorless, odorless gas
SOURCE AND USES: Produced during combustion of organic materials.
  Toxic byproduct of combustion.
TOXICITY: Cardiovascular toxicant (combines with hemoglobin)
SEE ALSO: Cellular sites of action   Ch. 4, p. 49
             Cardiovascular toxicology   Ch. 8, p. 110, 114
             Air pollution   Ch. 14, p. 202

CO

carbon monoxide

NAME: **Chlorofluorocarbons**
CHEMICAL FORMULA: CFC-11 CCl_3F, CFC-12 CCl_2F_2, CFC-113
  CCl_2FCClF_2
PHYSICAL PROPERTIES: Stable, nontoxic compounds
SOURCES AND USES: Synthetic chemicals used as refrigerants, propellants,
  among other uses.
TOXICITY: Nontoxic; influences health indirectly through damage to the
  ozone layer
SEE ALSO: Air pollution   Ch. 14, p. 206

CCl_3F	CFC-11
CCl_2F_2	CFC-12
CCl_2FCClF_2	CFC-113

NAME: **2,4-D; 2,4,5-T**
CHEMICAL FORMULA: 2,4-D(2,4-dichlorophenoxy) acetic acid) $C_8H_6Cl_2O_3$
  2,4,5-T (2,4,5-trichlorophenoxy) acetic acid) $C_8H_5Cl_3O_3$
PHYSICAL PROPERTIES:
SOURCE AND USES: Synthetic herbicides
TOXICITY: Irritants. 2,4-D LD_{50} (rat, oral) 375 mg/kg; 2,4,5-T LD_{50} (rat, oral)
  500 mg/kg
SEE ALSO: Renal toxicity Ch. 11, p. 166
              Water pollution Ch. 15, p. 218

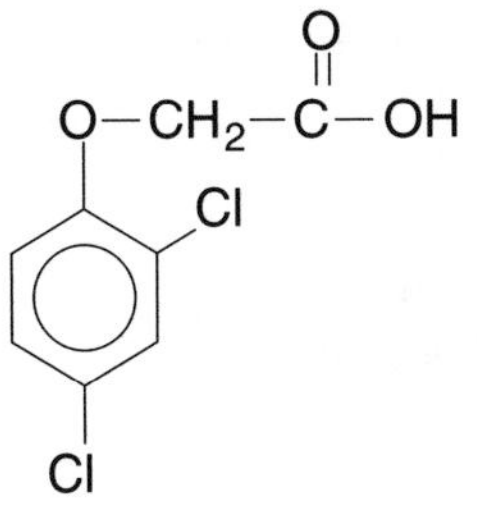

2,4-D
((2,4-dichlorophenoxy)acetic acid)

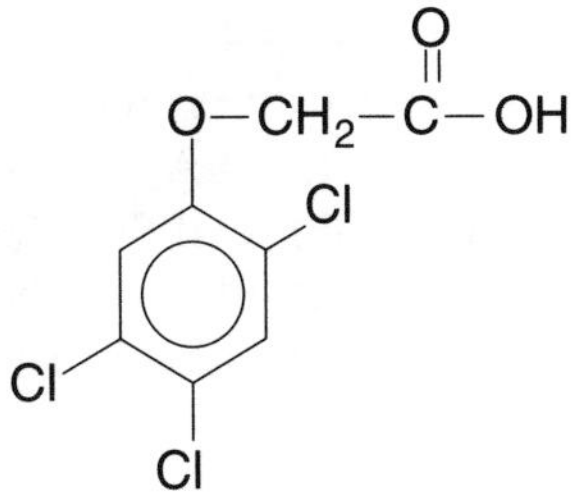

2,4.5-T
((2,4.5-trichlorophenoxy)acetic acid)

NAME: **Diethylstilbestrol (DES)**
CHEMICAL FORMULA: 4,4′-(1,2-diethyl-1,2ethenediyl)bisphenol $C_{18}H_{20}O_2$
PHYSICAL PROPERTIES:
SOURCE AND USES: Synthetic compound with estrogenic activity. Used at one
  time in prevention of miscarriage; also used in livestock feed to promote growth.
TOXICITY: Carcinogen
SEE ALSO: Reproductive toxicology
              and teratogenesis Ch. 6, p. 82

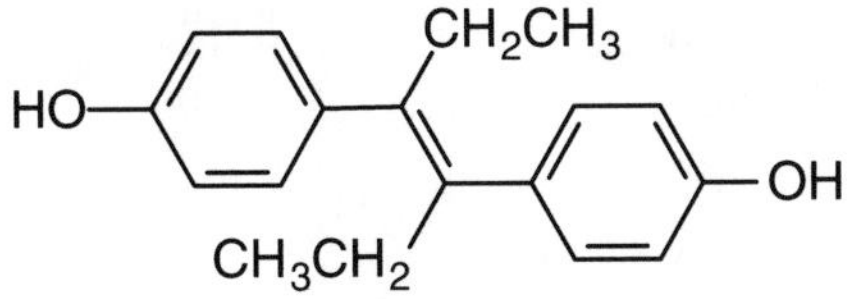

diethylstilbestrol

NAME: **Ethanol**
CHEMICAL FORMULA: C_2H_6O
PHYSICAL PROPERTIES: Colorless liquid
SOURCE AND USES: Produced through the process of fermentation. Used as
  recreational drug, as solvent in foods and medicines, and as industrial solvent.

TOXICITY: Acute exposures lead to nervous system depression; chronic exposures
lead to increased risks of neurologic and hepatic disease. Carcinogen, teratogen.

SEE ALSO: Reproductive toxicology
and teratology   Ch. 6, p. 82
Neurotoxicology   Ch. 9, p. 143
Hepatotoxicity   Ch. 10, p. 155

$$CH_3OH$$

ethanol

NAME: **Ethylene dibromide (EDB)**
CHEMICAL FORMULA: 1,2-dibromoethane $C_2H_4Br_2$
PHYSICAL PROPERTIES: Heavy liquid
SOURCES AND USES: Synthetic, used as fumigant
TOXICITY: Carcinogen, hepatotoxicant, nephrotoxicant

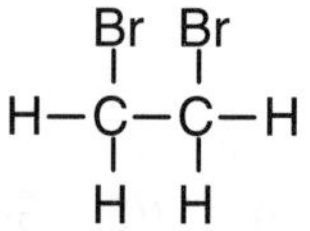

$$\begin{array}{cc} Br & Br \\ | & | \\ H-C-C-H \\ | & | \\ H & H \end{array}$$

EDB
1,2-dibromoethane

NAME: **Formaldehyde**
CHEMICAL FORMULA: CH_2O
PHYSICAL PROPERTIES: Colorless irritant gas
SOURCE AND USES: Byproduct of combustion, also manufactured syntheti-
cally. Used in production of resins, textiles, particle board and other products.
TOXICITY: Respiratory irritant, possible carcinogen
SEE ALSO: Respiratory toxicology   Ch. 7, p. 96
Immunotoxicology   Ch. 12, p. 177
Air pollution   Ch. 14, p. 206

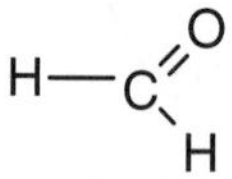

$$H-C{\overset{\displaystyle O}{\underset{\displaystyle H}{<}}}$$

formaldehyde

NAME: **Halogenated hydrocarbon solvents**
CHEMICAL FORMULAS: Carbon tetrachloride CCl_4
Chloroform $CHCl_3$

Dichloromethane CH$_2$Cl$_2$
Trichloroethylene C$_2$HCl$_3$

PHYSICAL PROPERTIES: Colorless, heavy liquids

SOURCE AND USES: Synthesized. Used as industrial solvents, cleaners, in synthesis of many organic compounds.

TOXICITY: Neurotoxic, hepatotoxic, toxic to cardiovascular and renal systems, carcinogenic

SEE ALSO: Biotransformation   Ch. 3, p. 32

```
            Cl
            |
  Cl —— C—Cl
            |
            Cl
```

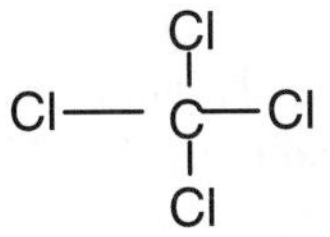

carbon tetrachloride

NAME: **Lead**

CHEMICAL FORMULA: Pb

PHYSICAL PROPERTIES: Heavy metal, also may form organolead compounds

SOURCE AND USES: Naturally occurring. Used in manufacture of alloys, batteries, pipes, pigments, and many other products.

TOXICITY: Neurotoxic, reproductive toxin

SEE ALSO: Reproductive toxicology

Pb

lead

NAME: **Mercury**

CHEMICAL FORMULA: Hg

PHYSICAL PROPERTIES: Heavy metal, also may form organomercury compounds

SOURCE AND USES: Naturally occurring

TOXICITY: Teratogenic, neurotoxicant, renal toxicant, irritant

SEE ALSO: Reproductive toxicity
                        and teratology   Ch. 6, p. 83
                 Neurotoxicology   Ch. 9, p. 142
                 Renal toxicity   Ch. 11, p. 165
                 Water pollution   Ch. 15, p. 222

$$CH_3\text{-}Hg^{\oplus}$$

methyl mercury

NAME: **Nitrates, nitrites**
CHEMICAL FORMULA: xNO_3, xNO_2
PHYSICAL PROPERTIES: Usually white or yellow powder or granules
SOURCE AND USES: Occur naturally. Used in manufacturing, preservation of
   meats, and fertilizers.
TOXICITY: Cardiovascular toxicant, possible role in carcinogenesis. LD_{50} for
   sodium nitrate (rabbits, oral) 2 g/kg; for sodium nitrite (rat, oral) 180 mg/kg
SEE ALSO: Cellular sites of action   Ch. 4, p. 50
                 Cardiovascular toxicology   Ch. 8, p. 111, 115
                 Water pollution   Ch. 15, p. 221

$$NaNO_2$$

sodium nitrite

$$NaNO_3$$

sodium nitrate

NAME: **Nitrogen dioxide**
CHEMICAL FORMULA: NO_2
PHYSICAL PROPERTIES: Irritant gas
SOURCE AND USES: Byproduct of combustion
TOXICITY: Respiratory toxicant
SEE ALSO: Respiratory toxicology   Ch. 7, p. 97
                 Air pollution   Ch. 14, p. 204

$$NO_2$$

nitrogen dioxide

NAME: **Organochlorine pesticides**
CHEMICAL FORMULA: DDT (dichlorodiphenyltrichloroethane) $C_{14}H_9Cl_5$

Chlordane (1,2,4,5,6,7,8,8-octochloro-2,3,3a,4,7,7a
-hexahydro-4,7-methano-1H-indene) $C_{10}H_6Cl_8$

Aldrin (1,2,3,4,10,10-hexachloro-1,4,4a,5,8,8a- hexa-
hydro-1,4:5,8-dimethanonaphthalene) $C_{12}H_8Cl_6$

Dieldrin (3,4,5,6,9,9-hexachloro-1a,2,2a,3,6,6a,7,7a -
octahydro-2,7:3,6-dimethanonapth[2,3-b]oxirene)
$C_{12}H_8Cl_6O$

Mirex (1,1a,2,2,3,3a,4,5,5,5a,5b,6-Dodecachloro-
octahydro-1,3,4-metheno-1H-cyclobuta[cd]pen-
talene) $C_{10}Cl_{12}$

Chlordecone (Kepone)(Decachlorooctahydro-1,3,4-
metheno-2H-cyclobuta[cd]pentalen-2-one) C_{10}
$Cl_{10}O$

PHYSICAL PROPERTIES: Crystals, insoluble in water
SOURCE AND USES: Synthetic insecticides, persistant in the environment
TOXICITY: Neurotoxic, chronic exposure may lead to hepatotoxicity. LD_{50} DDT

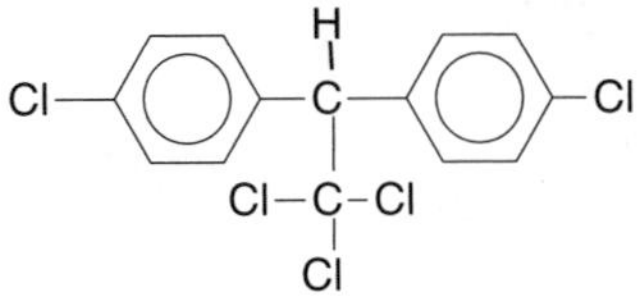

DDT
dichlorodiphenyltrichloroethane

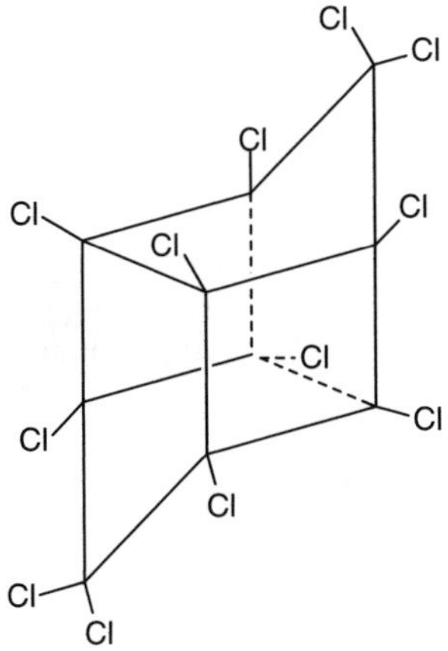

mirex

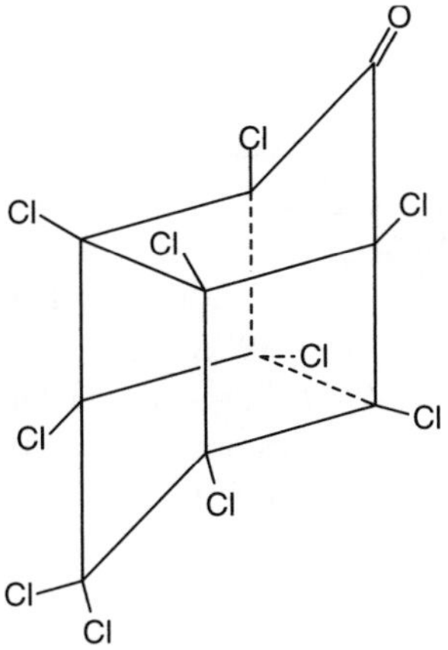

chlordecone
(Kepone®)

(human) 500 mg/kg, Chlordane (rat, ip) 343 mg/kg, Aldrin (rats, oral) 30 to 60 mg/kg, Dieldrin (rat, oral) 46 mg/kg; Mirex (rat, oral) 600 mg/kg, Chlordecone (rat, oral) 125 mg/kg

SEE ALSO: Water pollution   Ch. 15, p. 216

NAME: **Organophosphates**
CHEMICAL FORMULA: Parathion (phosphorothioic acid O,O-diethyl O-(4-
                                    nitrophenyl) ester) $C_{10}H_{14}NO_5PS$
                              Malathion ([(dimethoxypnosphinothioyl)thio]buta-
                                    nedioic acid diethyl ester) $C_{10}H_{19}O6PS_2$
PHYSICAL PROPERTIES: Pale liquid
SOURCE AND USES: Synthetic insecticide
TOXICITY: Neurotoxicants. Parathion LD_{50} (rat, oral) 3 to 10 mg/kg, Malathion LD_{50} (rat, oral) 1000 to 1400 mg/kg
SEE ALSO: Biotransformation   Ch. 2, p. 24
                   Cellular sites of action   Ch. 4. p. 39
                   Neurotoxicology   Ch. 9, pp. 134, 137
                   Water pollution   Ch. 15, p. 217

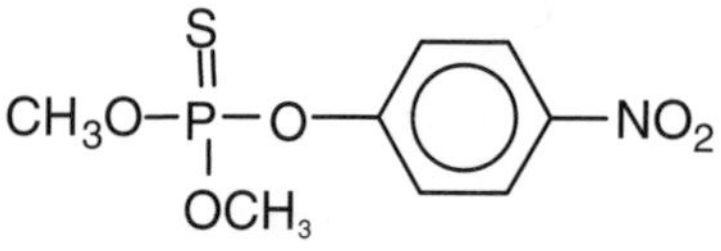

methyl parathion

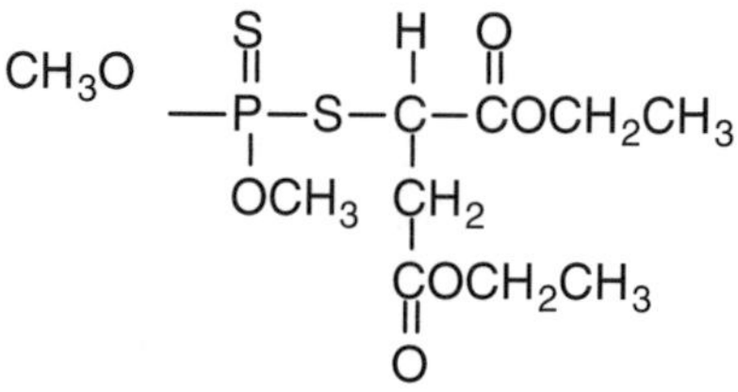

malathion

NAME: **Ozone**
CHEMICAL FORMULA: O_3
PHYSICAL PROPERTIES: Irritant gas
SOURCE AND USES: Produced as a byproduct of combustion, air pollutant
TOXICITY: Respiratory irritant
SEE ALSO: Respiratory toxicity   Chp. 7, p. 97
                   Air pollution   Chp. 14, p. 206

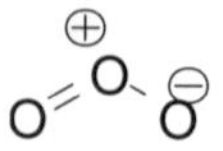

ozone

NAME: **Paraquat**

CHEMICAL FORMULA: 1,1'-dimethyl-4,4'-bipyridinium, $[C_{12}H_{14}N_2]^{2+}$

PHYSICAL PROPERTIES: Crystals

SOURCE AND USES: Synthetic herbicide

TOXICITY: Irritant, respiratory toxicant

SEE ALSO: Respiratory toxicity   Ch. 7, p. 97

            Water pollution   Ch. 15, p. 218

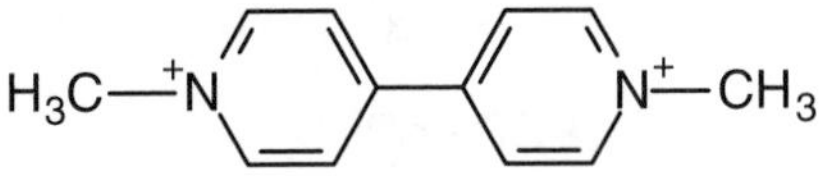

paraquat

NAME: **Petroleum products**

CHEMICAL FORMULA: Mixture of aliphatic and cyclic hydrocarbons, some aromatic hydrocarbons and other compounds

PHYSICAL PROPERTIES: Oily liquid

SOURCE AND USES: Naturally occurring. Petroleum or "crude oil" is distilled and separated into components which are typically used for fuels or lubricants.

TOXICITY: Some components are neurotoxic, others are potentially carcinogenic

SEE ALSO: Water pollution   Ch. 15, p. 213

petroleum components:

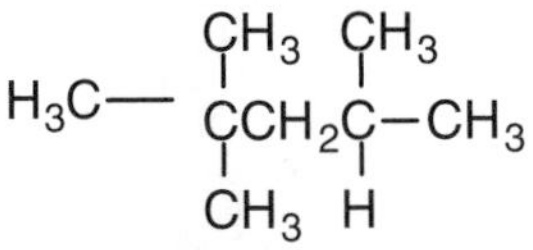

isoctane
(2.2,4-trimethylpentate)

H_3CCH_3

ethane

$CH_3CH_2CH_2CH_2CH_2CH_2CH_3$

n-heptane

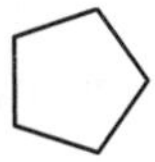

cyclopentane

NAME: **Polychlorinated biphenyls (PCBs)** and **polybrominated biphenyls (PBBs)**

CHEMICAL FORMULA: C_{12} with varying amounts of H and Cl

PHYSICAL PROPERTIES: Usually liquids

SOURCE AND USES: Synthetic compounds used in manufacture of electrical equipment

TOXICITY: Hepatotoxic, immunotoxic, potential carcinogens. PCBs LD_{50} (rat, oral) 1500 mg/kg.

SEE ALSO: Immunotoxicology   Ch. 15, p. 179
            Water pollution   Ch. 15, p. 219

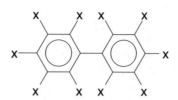

PCB or PBB
(polychlorinatedbiphenyl; x=Cl)
(polybrominatedbiphenyl; x=Br)

NAME: **Polycyclic aromatic hydrocarbons**
CHEMICAL FORMULA: Anthracene $C_{14}H_{10}$
                    Benzo[a]pyrene $C_{20}H_{12}$
                    3-methylcholanthrene (3-MC) $C_{21}H_{16}$
PHYSICAL PROPERTIES: Clear or yellowish powder
SOURCE AND USES: Produced during incomplete combustion of organic
   materials.
TOXICITY: Carcinogenic
SEE ALSO: Carcinogenesis   Ch. 5, p. 59
            Reproductive toxicology   Ch. 6, p. 77

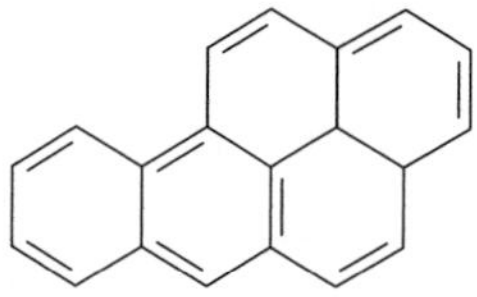

polycyclic aromatic hydrocarbon

H_3C

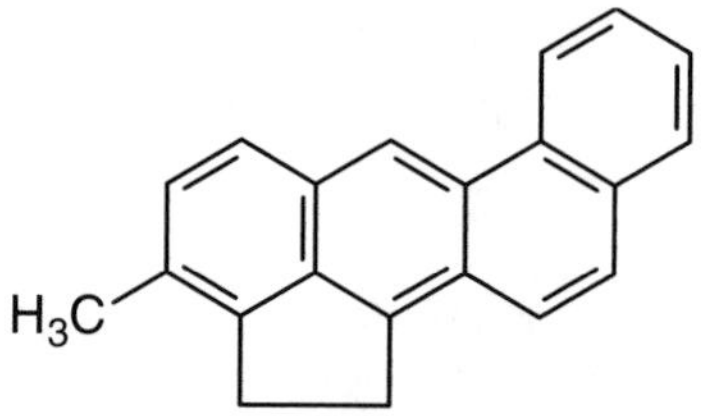

3-methylcholanthrene

NAME: **Pyrethroids**
CHEMICAL FORMULA: Allethrin (2,2-dimethyl-3-(2-methyl-1-propenyl)
                    cyclopropanecarboxylic acid 2-methyl-4-oxo-3-
                    (2-propenyl)-2- cyclopenten-1-yl ester) $C_{19}H_{26}O_3$
                    Permethrin (3-(2,2-dichloroethenyl)-2,2-dimethyl-
                    cyclopropanecarboxylic acid (3-phenoxyphenyl)
                    methyl ester) $C_{21}H_{20}Cl_2O_3$
                    Cypermethrin is the α-cyano derivative of Permethrin
PHYSICAL PROPERTIES: Liquid

SOURCE AND USES: Synthetic insecticide
TOXICITY: Neurotoxic
SEE ALSO: Neurotoxicology Ch. 9, p. 125

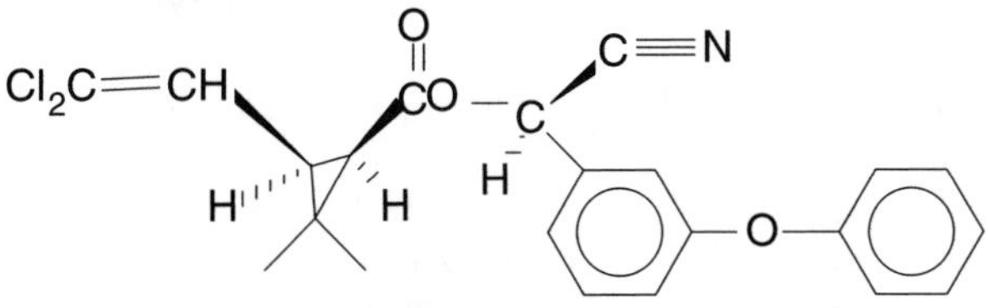

cypermethrin

NAME: **Sulfur dioxide**
CHEMICAL FORMULA: SO_2
PHYSICAL PROPERTIES: Irritant gas
SOURCE AND USES: Byproduct of combustion
TOXICITY: Respiratory irritant
SEE ALSO: Respiratory toxicology Ch. 7, p. 96
　　　　　　Air pollution Ch. 14, p. 204

$$SO_2$$

sulfur dioxide

NAME: **Tetrachlorodibenzodioxin (TCDD)**
CHEMICAL FORMULA: 2,3,7,8-tetrachlorodibenzo[b,e][1,4]dioxin $C_{12}H_4Cl_4O_2$
PHYSICAL PROPERTIES:
SOURCE: Contaminant formed during manufacture of certain herbicides
TOXICITY: Hepatotoxic, immunotoxic, teratogenic, carcinogenic. LD_{50}- (rat, oral) 0.02 to 0.04 mg/kg.
SEE ALSO: Biotransformation Ch. 3, p. 28
　　　　　　Carcinogenesis Ch. 5, p. 59
　　　　　　Immunotoxicity Ch. 12, p. 179
　　　　　　Water pollution Ch. 15, p. 218

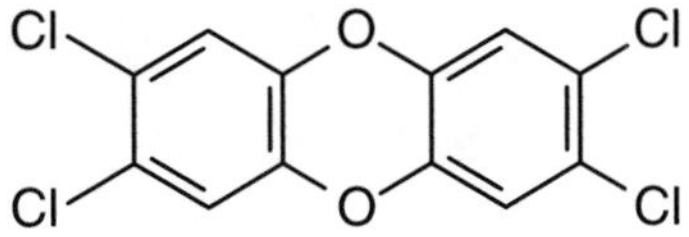

TCDD
(2,4,7,8-tetrachlorodibenzodioxin)

NAME: **Tetrodotoxin (TTX), saxitoxin (STX)**
CHEMICAL FORMULA: TTX $C_{11}H_{17}N_3O_8$; STX $[C_{10}H_{17}N_7O_4]^{2+}$
PHYSICAL PROPERTIES:
SOURCES AND USES: Naturally occurring toxins produced by fish (TTX)
  and dinoflagellates (STX).
TOXICITY: Neurotoxic. TTX LD_{50} (mice, ip) 10 $\mu g/kg$; STX LD_{50} (mice, oral)
  263 $\mu g/kg$.
SEE ALSO: Cellular sites of action   Ch. 4, p. 48
            Cardiovascular toxicology   Ch. 8, p. 106
            Neurotoxicology   Ch. 9, p. 123

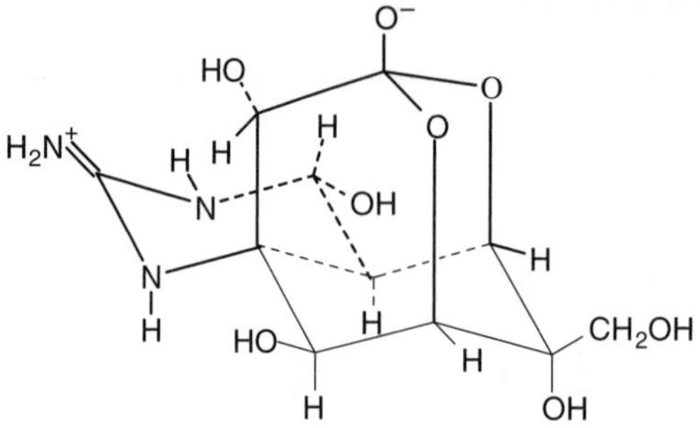

tetrodotoxin

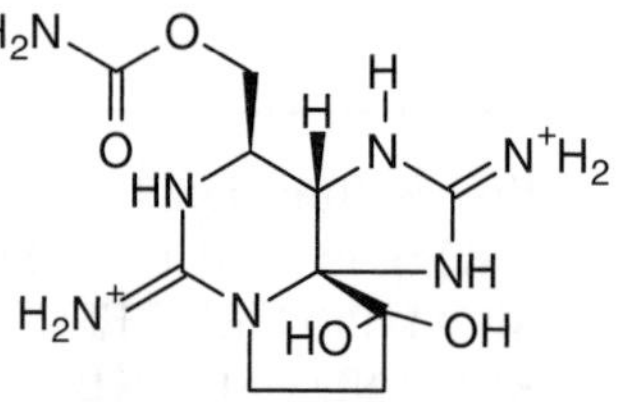

saxitoxin

NAME: **Thalidomide**
CHEMICAL FORMULA: 2-(2,6-dioxo-3-piperidinyl)-1H-isoindole-1,3(2H)-
  dione $C_{13}H_{10}N_2O_4$
PHYSICAL PROPERTIES:
SOURCE AND USES: Synthetic drug used to treat morning sickness.
TOXICITY: Teratogen
SEE ALSO: Reproductive toxicology and teratogenicity   Ch. 6, p. 81

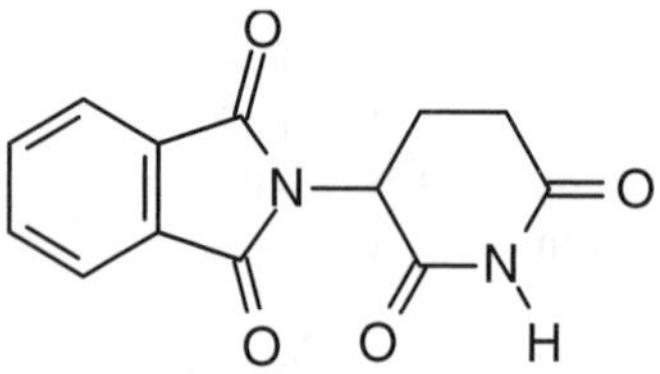

thalidomide

NAME: **Tobacco**
CHEMICAL FORMULA: Complex mixture of compounds including poly-
cyclic aromatic hydrocarbons, phenols, nicotine, nitrosamines
PHYSICAL PROPERTIES:
SOURCE AND USES: Tobacco plant, recreational use (smoking)
TOXICITY: Respiratory toxicant, carcinogenic
SEE ALSO: Respiratory toxicology   Ch. 7, p. 99

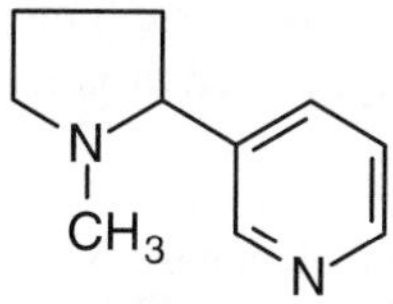

nicotine

NAME: **Toluene diisocyanate**
CHEMICAL FORMULA: 2,4-diisocyanatotoluene $C_9H_6N_2O_2$
PHYSICAL PROPERTIES: Liquid
SOURCE AND USES: Synthetic compound used in manufacturing
TOXICITY: Respiratory toxicant, immunotoxic
SEE ALSO: Respiratory toxicology   Ch. 7, p. 98
         Immunotoxicology   Ch. 12, p. 176

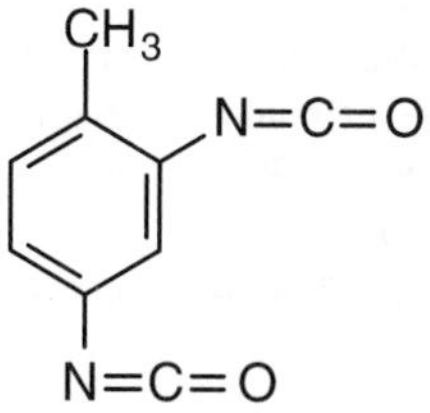

toluene 2,4-diisocyanate

REFERENCES

Most toxicity data in this appendix was derived from the same sources as cited in the chapters on that subject. Physical data, chemical data, and some LD_{50} figures were obtained from Windholz, M., Budavari S., Blumetti, R. F., and Otterbein, E. S., Eds., *Merck Index*, 10th ed., Merck and Co., In., Rahway, WJ, 1983.

The following books are textbooks which would serve as good general references for background information on basic biology, biochemistry, cell biology, anatomy and physiology, ecology, and environmental science.

Berne, R. M. and Levy, M. N., *Physiology,* C.V. Mosby, St. Louis, 1988.

Campbell, N. A., *Biology,* Benjamin Cummings, Menlo Park, CA, 1987.

Curtis, H. and Barnes, N. S., *Biology,* 5th ed., Worth Publishers, New York, 1989.

Guyton, A. C., *Textbook of Medical Physiology,* W. B. Saunders, Philadelphia, 1986.

Hole, J. W., Jr., *Human Anatomy and Physiology,* 6th ed., Wm. C. Brown, Dubuque, IA, 1993.

Kaufman, D. G. and Franz, C. M., *Biosphere 2000. Protecting our Global Environment,* HarperCollins, New York, 1993.

Martini, F., *Fundamentals of Anatomy and Physiology,* Prentice Hall, Englewood Cliffs, NJ, 1992.

Miller, G. T., Jr., *Living in the Environment,* Wadsworth, Belmont, CA, 1992.

Morgan, M. D., Moran, J. M., and Wiersma, J. H., *Environmental Science. Managing Biological and Physical Resources,* Wm. C. Brown, Dubuque, IA, 1993.

Smith, R. L., *Elements of Ecology,* 3rd ed., Harper Collins, New York, 1992.

Spence, A. P. and Mason, E. B., *Human Anatomy and Physiology,* 4th ed., West Publishing, St Paul, MN, 1992.

Stiling, P., *Introductory Ecology,* Prentice Hall, Englewood Cliffs, NJ, 1992.

Stryer, L. *Biochemistry,* W. H. Freeman and Company, New York, 1988.

Tortora, G. J. and Grabowski, S. R., *Principles of Anatomy and Physiology,* 7th ed., Harper & Row, New York, 1993.

Wolfe, S. L., *Molecular and Cellular Biology,* Wadsworth, Belmont, CA, 1993.

INDEX